The Barrett's Diet Plan

"Change your life!"

Groundbreaking 14-day diet plan with recipes that will change the way you eat, look, and feel forever!

Table of Contents

1. Introduction..1

2. Message.....................................17

3. The Plan......................................18

4. The Rules...............................21

5. Plant Based and Organic Foods.......22

6. Tips and Suggestions.....................23

7. Freestyle Snacks............................25

8. Kitchen Items and Tools.................28

9. Recipe Guidelines..........................29

10. Shopping Tips...............................30

11. 62 Recipes....................................31

12. Food Buying Tips and Guidelines.....163

13. Food Labeling................................179

14. Food Label Glossary.......................187

15. References....................................251

Introduction

As a restaurant owner, caterer and lifelong restaurant industry worker I have been in and around kitchens and food for my entire adult life. I have spent thousands of hours interacting with people who are around me for one reason, to eat. Not only in restaurants and catering halls but also in people's homes and backyards when catering private events. I have spent countless hours in the private kitchens of people, observing how and what people eat. I have seen the contents of their cupboards and refrigerators. I have also listened to a wide array of diet fads, food trends and heath restrictions that customers have requested during my career. The one consistent habit that I have observed over the last thirty years is that most of us are simply unhealthy and inconsistent eaters. Yes, I include my past self in that observation. I have observed a shift, however over the last decade. There is much more focus on unprocessed and whole foods. Organic and sustainable foods are now a mainstay in many communities. Terms like "slow food", "clean eating" and "farm to table" are now common terms in mainstream media. It is a good sign that this new trend in our diets has the attention of the media. Our knowledge base as a nation has greatly increased thanks to social media. These diet practices are not fads, they are manifestations of the vast amount of food knowledge we have gained as a better informed nation. The advertising media and the FDA are no longer our main sources for our food knowledge. We are no longer solely informed by advertisements and force fed false information by the government. Look back at old tobacco ads, sugar ads, and dairy ads. All of us believed milk was the healthiest possible thing we could ingest. Drink your milk! This information was forced upon us by the dairy industry who paid experts to lobby the government. Healthy guidelines showed up in schools telling us to drink our milk and eat more beef. Today, we are experiencing a change in the narrative. It is now common knowledge that processed foods and meats are laden with antibiotics, chemical additives, and GMO's. Over Processing of food has stripped the nutrients out and increased the density of the harmful components in our food. By appealing to the addictive nature of our palettes the food industry has fueled the obesity epidemic in this country. We are now informed that too much sugar, dairy, red meat, processed foods, soft drinks and alcohol are the leading causes of many of the diseases that are killing us today. Obesity is now an actual epidemic. Our healthcare system is completely bogged down with costs related to diabetes and heart disease both deadly conditions attributable to obesity.

Our busy lives have forced us to constantly feel rushed and tend to eat more snack food, processed food, and sweets. Since the 1950's we have produced and promoted foods that are fast and easy. "Grab and go". "Fast food". "Comfort food". Families who had nightly dinners now had only Sunday dinners because everyone was getting busier and busier. Our food products became quicker and cheaper and easier to prepare. Microwave cooking and processed frozen dinners were time savers. The advertising industry was well aware of this and knew how to sell it by appealing to the busy nature of our lives.

Today, In the U.S. we talk about dieting more than anyone else in the world but as a whole, we are gluttons. Europeans, Asians, and pretty much all other cultures eat with purpose, with attention to timing and portions, and types of foods based on daily life-cycles. Whole foods are the norm. Sustainability is commonplace in other countries. We are a nation of immigrants and it has become a national tradition to eat foods from all over the world and to have access to many diverse and cultural eating habits. This is one of the greatest things about our country but we all fell into the trap of eating it all, all the time, as fast as we can. In America, we eat anything and everything all the time. There is such an abundance of food and so many different types of food that we have created new ways to eat it all. We combine it all together in sandwiches, pizzas, omelettes, buffets. Just think about how the microwave impacted our culture. We now could eat all this food in a fraction of the time. With all the added chemicals and preservatives and sugar our body does not even know it is full. We just cram it in. If there is a way to get more food into our bodies, it seems that America has a solution. In other words, we are gluttons, true gluttons. Gluttony, defined as habitual greed or excess in eating. All anyone needs to do is to look at the average body shape of middle class americans in any shopping mall across the country. There, you will see firsthand the results of our gluttonous eating habits.

According the National Center for Health, 68% of U.S. adults over the age of 20 are considered overweight or obese.

Obesity Statistics for Adults Age 20 and Older in the United States

- More than two-thirds (68.8 percent) of adults are considered to be overweight or obese.

- More than one-third (35.7 percent) of adults are considered to be obese.

- More than 1 in 20 (6.3 percent) have extreme obesity.

- Almost 3 in 4 men (74 percent) are considered to be overweight or obese.

- The prevalence of obesity is similar for both men and women (about 36 percent).

- About 8 percent of women are considered to have extreme obesity.

My own personal eating habits were terrible when I was younger. I too was a glutton. Not only a glutton for food but a glutton for punishment as well. The food I ate caused me pain and discomfort, always. Working in fine dining restaurants, I had access to the best foods, all the time. In fact, for the last 25 years I have had the honor of having almost all of my meals prepared by chefs in commercial kitchens. Considering that I always worked 60-70 hour weeks that is almost every meal! Sounds like a luxurious perk, but the late hours, constant snacking on rich, sugar and fat laden foods, all took their toll on my health. Working in restaurants my go-to dinner was usually red meat, mashed potatoes, some ice cream for dessert and a few beers to wash it all down. I ate like a king as the saying goes. My daily eating habits weren't much better. I ate fried foods, processed meats,lots of soda, lots of dairy. I would easily drink a quart of milk and 2 liters of soda daily. Looking back now I realize that all of my discomfort and bloating and gastric distress was caused by the types of foods I ate and the timing of my meals. Fried foods, fatty foods, meat, dairy are all enemies to a healthy diet regimen. All of my sedentary moments were occupied by severe heartburn and constant gastric distress. I would awake at night and vomit. Often, I would wake up choking on bile which was the result of me laying down prior to completely digesting my food. The foods that my body was struggling to digest were incredibly complex and required more acid production thus leading to severe heartburn. I also suffered severe pains in my lower abdomen. Often I would be in such distress I would pass out in the bathroom. I was seriously prone to acid reflux and was lucky because it was the nineties and the drug companies had come out with something to mask all of these bad symptoms related to eating all that rich, sugar laden, hard-to-digest food.

Behold the dawn of prescription antacids clinically known as proton pump inhibitors or PPIs. Evidence emerged by the end of the 1970s that the newly discovered proton pump (H^+/K^+ ATPase) in the secretory membrane of the parietal cell was the final step in acid secretion. Drug companies were now able to produce drugs inhibiting the production of acid in the body. As a result of such optimization the first proton pump inhibiting drug was released on the market, omeprazole. Other PPIs like lansoprazole and pantoprazole would follow in its footsteps, claiming their share of a flourishing market.

Basically, the FDA should have just call these drugs "things to mask the symptoms while you slowly die". In 2010 the FDA issued a dire warning on proton pump inhibitors. Healthcare professionals and users of proton pump inhibitors should be aware of the possible increased risk of fractures of the hip, wrist, and spine with the use of proton pump inhibitors, and weigh the known benefits against the potential risks when deciding to use them. Food Blogger, Chris Kresser wrote about this FDA report and stated "In a rare instance of the FDA actually doing its job, a report was issued on Tuesday cautioning against the prolonged use of a class of acid stopping drugs called proton-pump inhibitors (PPIs). Who knows, maybe someone at the FDA read my series on heartburn and GERD, especially this article and this one detailing the dangers of acid stopping drugs? This is a really big deal. PPIs are one of the most popular classes of drugs prescribed. Doctors wrote 114 million prescriptions for them last year. Americans spend $5.1 billion on Nexium, the most popular

PPI, alone. The FDA report cautions against high doses or prolonged use of PPIs, because they've been shown to increase the risk of infection, bone fractures and dementia. But the danger doesn't stop there. As I pointed out in my series, all acid stopping drugs (not just PPIs) inhibit nutrient absorption, promote bacterial overgrowth, reduce resistance to infection and increase the risk of cancer and other serious diseases. So, in review, these FDA approved hartburn preventing drugs contain the following risks:

- Decrease in bone density
- Inhibit nutrient absorption
- Increase bacterial Overgrowth
- Reduce resistance to infections
- Increase risk of cancer and numerous other diseases

I, along with hundreds of thousands of other americans began taking one of these acid reducing pills called prevacid. I could eat anything and not "feel the burn", heartburn. The problem with these drugs is that they MASK the symptoms. The damage is still being done to your body but you simply don't feel the symptoms. That is how the drug was designed. Not a cure, simply a mask, a diversion. We see television and Internet ads heartburn relief followed by ads for chicken wings and sugar cereals and 2-for-1 appetizers at the local restaurant. Take a pill, eat more! Should be our national slogan. This is our American diet, eat whatever you want and just take a pill if you have any problems. This is one of the primary reasons that healthcare costs are so high in the United States. I am not a fan of taxing people for sugar consumption but I can certainly understand the logic from an economic standpoint. We allow these horribly unhealthy products to be sold and then the healthcare industry and the government bears the brunt of the costs related to treating all of the heath issues they caused.

A sad parallel is the fact that in the last 20 years as these antacids became so popular, esophageal cancer incidences began to rise. Esophageal Cancer is now the leading cancer among white males ages 35-45. Esophageal Cancer is 8th on the list of most deadly cancers according to *The American Cancer Society.*

Until the 1970s, the most common type of esophageal cancer in the United States was squamous cell carcinoma, which had smoking and alcohol consumption as the leading risk factors. Since then, there has been a steep increase in the incidence of esophageal adenocarcinoma, for which the most common predisposing factor is gastroesophageal reflux disease (GERD).

The incidence of a certain type of esophageal cancer called esophageal adenocarcinoma is rising faster than that of any other cancer in the United States, according to research studies performed at the National Institutes of Health. Once diagnosed, the prognosis for esophageal adenocarcinoma is poor, with only approximately 13 percent of patients surviving five years from the time of diagnosis. One reason is that the cancer is usually diagnosed at an advanced stage. Unless a patient is monitored regularly by endoscopy, esophageal cancer may not be detected unless a tumor has grown large enough to obstruct the esophagus. That's why regular monitoring for patients with a syndrome called Barrett's Esophagus is so important because steps can be taken to prevent the symptoms from progressing into cancer.

My epiphany regarding healthy eating and the basis for research behind this book came as a result of a series of gastroenterological tests and my experiences that followed. I was 36 years old and married with two children. I had been suffering from severe heartburn since I was a teenager and dulled the symptoms with antacids. After so many years of postponing doctor visits it was recommended that I go for advanced testing because I was in such constant pain and distress. After being hospitalized for severe pain hours after eating a corned beef dinner on St. Patrick's Day, I was sent for an endoscopy procedure which is a full camera scope of the esophagus. It was then that I was diagnosed with a condition called Barrett's Esophagus.

Barrett's is defined in Wikipedia as Barrett's Esophagus , sometimes called Barrett Syndrome. Barrett's esophagus refers to an abnormal change in the cells of the lower portion of the esophagus. It is characterized by the replacement of the normal stratified squamous epithelium lining of the esophagus by simple columnar epithelium with goblet cells (which are usually found lower in the gastrointestinal tract). The medical significance of Barrett's esophagus is the strong association (about 0.5% per patient-year) with esophageal adenocarcinoma, an often deadly cancer, because of which it is considered to be a premalignant condition.

The main cause of Barrett's esophagus is thought to be an adaptation to chronic acid exposure from reflux esophagitis. The incidence of esophageal adenocarcinoma has increased substantially in the Western world in recent years. The condition is found in 5–15% of patients who seek medical care for heartburn (gastroesophageal reflux disease), although a large subgroup of patients with Barrett's esophagus do not have symptoms. Diagnosis requires endoscopy (more specifically, esophagogastroduodenoscopy, a procedure in which a fibre optic cable is inserted through the mouth to examine the esophagus, stomach, and duodenum) and biopsy. The cells of Barrett's esophagus, after biopsy, are classified into four general categories: nondysplastic, low-grade dysplasia, high-grade dysplasia, and frank carcinoma. High-grade dysplasia and early stages of adenocarcinoma can be treated by endoscopic resection and new endoscopic therapies such as radiofrequency ablation, whereas advanced stages (submucosal) are generally advised to undergo surgical treatment. Nondysplastic and low-grade patients are generally advised to undergo annual observation with endoscopy, with radiofrequency ablation as a therapeutic option. In high-grade dysplasia, the risk of developing cancer might be at 10% per patient-year or greater. The condition is named after the Australian-born British thoracic surgeon Norman Barrett (1903–1979), who described it in 1950. Development of *Barrett's Esophagus* is the worst case scenario before cancer for sufferers of reflux. It is non-reversible but maintainable with strict diet and lifestyle changes.

I was concerned but very matter of fact about the whole issue. I am a very concrete person. At least I knew what it was and what I needed to do,so I thought. The doctor had a talk with me and said, "Hey, you're young. You're probably not going to develop cancer but this is the easiest diet to cheat on and if you do not follow a healthy diet you probably will develop esophageal cancer and die." After all this, He handed me a single piece of paper with a diet for reflux patients and wished me luck.The diet stated some very basic guidelines:

- No tomatoes or tomato products
- Avoid fried foods
- Avoid alcohol and coffee
- Avoid carbonated beverages

- No citric acid

- Do not eat three hours before bed.

I had expected a more detailed diet. This was all good information but I thought to myself, there must be a better solution! There must be more information on how to reverse this condition.

As I started to discuss my condition with friends and family, I realized that few had heard of the condition. My financial advisor at the time had heard of it and knew it well. He told me of another client of his, the same age as me. This person was 35, diagnosed with Barrett's and ignored the advice of doctors. He decided to just keep taking the prescription antacid medicine as he did not feel the burning with the medication so he figured he would be fine. Within a year he had to have half of his esophagus removed. He was on a liquid diet for 6 months. In the hospital for a month. He said he did not feel like a human being for a year. This story scared me more than anything. Suddenly it became very real for me.

Now, armed with my culinary background and my newfound fear of developing esophageal cancer. I decided to create my own personal diet plan to give me peace of mind that I was doing the right thing and taking the right course of action.The diet plan that I created allowed me to lose 28 pounds in less than six months. I attained a massive increase in energy, eradicated any heartburn, Increased my libido and achieved better focus and overall mental clarity. I stopped taking the pills completely. I returned for another endoscopy exactly one year later and they found no indication of any inflammation or Barrett's Esophagus. Now, more than 14 years later I have kept the weight off and still have no sign of Barrett's condition. Following this diet resulted in losing 24% of my body weight as well as eradicating the symptoms of my Barrett's Syndrome. The doctor stated that the condition is irreversible but after 1 year a new endoscopy showed zero symptoms.

Message from Russ

Folks, this diet plan is designed to not only save your life but to enhance the vibrancy of your life. My poor diet habits and development of a rare precancerous condition led me to discover this amazing diet plan. It changed my life and I am confident it will change yours! You've already purchased the book but I will say it again, I will refund 100% of your money if you are not satisfied after following this diet plan for only 2 weeks. Now, the plan starts here. I wish you the best of luck. I am on your team. Email me at Russ@thebarrettsdiet.com ! Seriously, ask me anything, tell me your progress, send me before and after photos. I promise you, I will respond to every single email. YOU are my passion. I want YOU to be your best self and feel awesome every day. Now get to work! Start Eating for your life!

– Russ

The Plan

Welcome to the beginning of an incredible journey! Follow these steps I have outlined for you and I promise at bare minimum, you will feel awesome! Stay focused and use this book as a springboard for your own healthy lifestyle and you will reap the rewards for the rest of your life.

Your first step is to set aside an hour or two to create your personal plan. Only you know how to make this work best for you. You will need to shop for at least a week's worth of groceries based on the menu items you decide you want to eat during your fourteen days. Most clients plan out a 7-day period and mix it up with different menu items the second week. Think of this as your own personal restaurant menu for the next two weeks. Consult with your family, your partner, your spouse, your dog. Whoever may be impacted by what is in your fridge and in your cupboard should be on board with your diet plan. Many have actually used a separate fridge and a dedicated section of the cupboards for their own two-week plan. This may be a good idea if you have children. They most likely will not raid your healthy food. Another option is to get the whole household involved, we all know realistically this may not work but try it, who knows? From this point on you are in it! Start working the plan. Good luck! I am here to help if you need. Email me with any questions, I will reply. Enjoy the book, work the plan, change your life!

The 20 Rules

1. No more than 5 grams of refined or processed sugar per day
2. No carbonated beverages other than sparkling water.
3. Zero deep fried food or fatty oils (up to 2 ounces of real butter or peanut oil per day is allowed for sauteing).
4. Zero fruit juices
5. Eat only during a 10 hour waking window for 5 consecutive days weekly.
6. Only clear alcohol or wine. 1-2 glasses or cocktails per day
7. Zero white flour.
8. Only 1 meal of chicken or beef protein per week
9. Eat 3 main meals per day spaced at least 3 hours apart
10. Exercise for 30 minutes per day. Break a sweat.
11. Snack and follow recommended portion sizes
12. Consume 90% unprocessed foods. All original ingredients
13. Drink 8 oz water immediately upon waking
14. Only 1 large cup (up to 16 oz) of caffeinated coffee or tea per day
15. Drink, Drink, Drink Water. At least 64 oz water per day Stay hydrated!
16. Do not eat for at least three hours prior to going to sleep
17. No dairy other than allotted cheese. 3 slices or 4 oz of shredded cheese per day
18. No more than 20 grams of carbohydrates per day
19. Eat until you are full and then stop
20. Chew Your Food thoroughly, do not rush any meals.

Plant Based and Organic Foods

Most of the recipes in this book consist of plant based ingredients and whole organic foods. We incorporate a very limited amount of dairy as well as small amounts of lean meat and poultry. Meat and poultry is much harder for our bodies to digest. Only 1 meal per week of any lean, organic beef or chicken. A healthy digestive system is absolutely critical to a healthy lifestyle. Add 6-8 oz portions and no more than one meal per week. By lean meat we are referring to beef or poultry only, no fat, no skin, no cartilage. Ideally, we recommend an 80% plant based diet supplemented with 10% wild fish or seafood and 10% lean natural beef or poultry.

Organic can be slightly misleading. We recommend whole foods and original, unprocessed foods. You do not have to be 100% certified organic to lead a healthy lifestyle. It is a good goal but unnecessary to follow a healthy diet regimen.

Make it your goal to lead a primarily plant based diet while following our recommended guidelines.

Many long term studies have proven that a 100% plant based diet leads to longer lifespan and can eradicate diseases such as cancer and heart disease. Maintaining a purely plant based diet is challenging and not easily adopted by all. Supplementing with small amounts of fish and meat weekly allow you to have "cheat" days.

Tips and Suggestions

- The first 3-4 days are hard. Stay focused. Snack often.

- Read _all_ labels for ingredients. Get used to this practice.

- Stick to your favorite meals. It will be much easier and less shopping. You could choose 6-12 of the recipes in this book and just mix them up throughout the 14 days. You'll notice that you have leftover ingredients from many meals. Calculate how many other portions of those meals that you can make. You can pre-portions all or most ingredients for future meals to save you time.

- Basic cooking skills are needed. Any tips you need on how to saute, chop, dice, broil, bake, fry can all be found readily on youtube as well as on our website.

- Eat a lot of the freestyle cheat snacks. A snack means you eat something to curb the hunger you're feeling in between main meals. Eat the recommended portion of snacks. You'll find that you rarely crave more than the recommended portion. Watch the portions. Its best to pre-portion everything for at least a week at a time.

- Use 2 and 4 oz souffle cups with lids for measuring and portioning. USe pint and quart plastic deli containers.These can be purchased at any party or restaurant supply store. Take the time to portion things out and package them ahead of time. Using consistent sized containers will help you maintain proper portion sizes. Once we empty the food onto a plate, we all misjudge how many handfuls we've eaten!

- When shopping, try your best to purchase ALL original, natural ingredients. It does not have to be "certified" organic. Organic is always a good start but can be costly. Do your best to buy fresh, original ingredients. Shop locally at farm stands or green markets. Plan your meals as simply as possible. Nothing processed. Nothing in wrappers or cans.

- Put the plan in overdrive.
  - Stick to all plant based meals.
  - Go heavy on leafy greens and superfoods.
  - Extend 10 hour fasting window to 7 days
  - All other rules apply.

- Eating out at a restaurant? Plan ahead, check the menu. Stay away from any fast food restaurant. Best option is to order broiled fish with steamed vegetables. Request no butter or oil. It's hard not to snack and overeat. Do not go hungry, try to have a snack before you go to a restaurant.

- Be prepared. Have pre-portioned non-perishable snacks in your car at all times.

- Limit alcohol to only 1-2 drinks per day if at all. Stick to clear alcohol, red or white wine. No beer, mixers, sugary spirits.

- Condiments and sauces can be laden with sugar and chemicals. Use our recommended recipes for condiments or purchase vegan, sugar free condiments.

Freestyle Snacks

These are your go-to in between main meal snacks. Portions are key!

Baby Carrots - 4-6

Bananas - 1

Apples - 1

Peach - 1

Wasabi Peas - 4 oz

Raw Broccoli - 4 oz

Snap Peas - 4 oz

Smart Food - 4 oz

Natural Peanut Butter - 1 teaspoon

Kale Chips - 4 oz

Avocado - 1

Black Bean Chips - 4oz

Snap Peas - 4oz

Pickles - 1 whole pickle

Hummus - 4oz

Strawberries - 4oz

Raspberries - 4oz

Blackberries - 4oz

Raw Honey - 2oz

Salad with sugar free dressing - 6 oz

Blueberries 4oz

Broccoli 4oz

Oats ½ cup

Salmon (wild) 6oz

Soy 1oz

Spinach 4oz

Tea (green or black) 1

Walnuts 4oz

Almonds 4oz

Cashews 4oz

Yogurt 4oz

Kale 4oz

Sweet Potato 1

Apple 1

Banana 1

Cocoa 1oz

Quinoa ½ cupBlueberries 4oz

Greek Yogurt 4oz

Avocado 1

Natural Peanut Butter 4 oz

Coconut 4oz

Coconut Oil 2oz

Beets 4oz

Strawberries 4oz

Pumpkin 4oz

Butter 2oz

Walnuts 4oz

Almonds 4oz

Chia Seeds 1oz

Mustard Greens 4oz

Watermelon 4oz

Cranberries 4oz

Cauliflower 4oz

Leeks 4oz

Lentils 4oz

Grapefruit 4oz

Asparagus 4oz

Broccoli Rabe 6oz

Recommended kitchen items to have available:

- Small kitchen scale

- Sandwich Size Ziploc Bags for portion and storage

- 1 Gallon Zip-Loc bags for portion and storage

- Measuring cups and Bowls

- Plastic portion cups with lids (2 oz and 4oz)

- Deli containers with lids (pint and quart)

- Small inexpensive "pulsing" food processor.

Recipe Guidelines

- All foods must be real, hormone free, natural, original. They don't necessarily have to be certified organic but avoid any processed, GMO foods. Do not purchase anything pre-packaged, boxed, wrapped or canned.

- Use true free range eggs or organic egg whites.

- Follow portion sizes precisely.

- Check for sugar content and all ingredients. It's very easy to substitute something and wind up consuming a lot of sugar. Aim for zero added sugar!! Maximum total added sugar = 20 grams. Zero is best.

- All bread should be white flour free, ezekiel or true 100% whole grain or 100% whole wheat.

- Substituting your own recipes - Awesome, go for it! Just follow the rules. Send us your recipes so we can feature them on our blog!

Shopping Tips

- Take your time, make a list. Use your checklist!

- Do not buy anything other than what you will eat for the week.

- Don't shop for the family, shop for your diet. I'm not suggesting you ignore the family but make a separate trip for your diet. It will be hard but keep a section of the fridge just for you or if possible, use the garage fridge or the old college fridge you have laying around in storage.

- Plan out your meals <u>before</u> you go shopping.

- I will stress again and again. Choose wisely from the suggested list of dishes. Pick dishes that you think you will like. Unless you are a chef you probably won't have all 52 dishes listed in this book during your fourteen days. I want to hear about it if you do however, that would be awesome!!! The whole idea is to give you a wide range of options to choose from. We provide some popular healthy meals as recommendations but the Internet has thousands more. Jts follow the rules and guidelines.

Recipes

Breakfast

Meal #1	"The Great White Omelette"
Ingredients	2 Organic Egg Whites or 6 oz Organic liquid egg whites 1 Teaspoon of Butter 4 oz Baby Spinach 2 Slice Cheddar Cheese or 4 oz shredded 1 slice Ezekiel Bread
Substitutions	*Organic Eggs, Broccoli, Asparagus, Kale, Swiss, Gouda, Jack, American*
Shopping List	Organic Eggs or liquid egg whites; baby spinach, salted butter, shredded cheddar cheese, Ezekiel or Whole grain bread
Suggestions	Lots of good egg white products available
Preparation	Portion egg whites, spinach, and cheese
Cooking Instructions	Heat nonstick skillet, add butter (save a tiny bit for toast) and quickly swirl around entire pan; add spinach and cook until wilted. Add egg whites; gently push eggs to

	center of pan with rubber spatula until eggs begin to form. As soon as you can move entire circle of egg as one piece, flip to the other side. Add cheese. As cheese begins to melt fold omelette in half and plate. Toast slice of Ezekiel bread as as you are cooking an omelette.
Suggested Spice, Side or Condiment	Hot sauce, Homemade Salsa, Sugar Free Ketchup, Pepper

Meal #2	"Good Crunchy Morning"
Ingredients	Cereal of your choice (oats, flax,dried berries,granola, etc..) Watch the sugar content! 6 oz Almond Milk 4 oz Blueberries 1 Banana
Substitutions	*Any non-citrus fruit*
Shopping List	Cereal, Almond Milk, Blueberries, Bananas
Suggestions	Stick to plain almond milk
Suggested Spice, Side or Condiment	Honey

Meal #3	"Hot and Fruity"
Ingredients	Hot oats, bananas, apples, cranberries
Substitutions	*Have fun! Add Any citrus free fruit*
Shopping List	Oats, bananas, apples, cranberries
Suggestions	Look for oats with very little or zero sugar
Preparation	Chop one banana in ½ inch discs, core 1 apple and cut into ¼ inch cubes, 2 ounces fresh cranberries
Cooking Instructions	Boil 1 cup water with dash salt and add ½ cup oats. Cook 5 minutes
Suggested Spice, Side or Condiment	Real maple syrup, honey

1.

Meal #4	"Green Eggs Omelette"
Ingredients	Spinach, eggs, Avocado, mushrooms, butter
Substitutions	*Any green leafy vegetable, any mushroom variety. Eggs can be prepared any way and combined with these ingredients.*
Shopping List	Baby spinach, Avocado, free range eggs, medium mushrooms, butter
Suggestions	Have this often. It's a quick, easy, hot meal that will fill you up! The avocado replaces the cheese and still gives you the creamy texture.
Preparation	Scramble 2 eggs Chop 2 cups baby spinach 1 Avocado Sliced Chop 1 cup mushrooms Prepare 1 tablespoon butter
Cooking Instructions	Add butter to hot saute pan Coat pan with hot butter as it melts. Add mushrooms first, then add spinach directly to mushrooms while sauteing. Cook until spinach wilted. Pour scrambled eggs over the top. Gently push mixture to center of pan as liquid begins to harden. As soon as you can shake pan and all ingredients begin to slide as one, add avocado and flip to uncooked side and finish cooking for 2-3 minutes. Fold in half and plate.

Suggested Spice, Side or Condiment	Fresh Salsa, Sriracha, Salt, Pepper

Meal # 5	"Mañana Burrito"
Ingredients	Onion, green bell pepper, 8-inch whole grain tortilla, tofurkey sausage, cheese
Substitutions	*Tofurkey turkey, tofu or any vegetarian meat substitute, parsley, Any green cruciferous vegetable, fresh homemade salsa*
Shopping List	Organic eggs, Tofurkey sausages, onion, pepper, cilantro, whole grain wraps, olive oil
Suggestions	Vegetarian meat substitutes vary wildly in texture and quality. There are some horrible products out there that will make you want to go back to fatty meats! We recommend Tofurkey brand meat substitutes.
Preparation	1/2 tablespoon peanut oil 1/8 cup diced onion 1/8 cup diced red or orange bell pepper 1/4 cups diced Tofurkey sausage (fully cooked) 1/2 tablespoons finely chopped parsley or cilantro 2 free range eggs, lightly beaten

	1/4 cup shredded pepper jack cheese
	1 (8-inch) organic whole-grain tortillas
Cooking Instructions	1. In a large skillet, heat oil over medium heat. Add onion and bell pepper and cook, stirring, for 4 to 5 minutes or until veggies are tender. Add tofurkey sausage and cook 1 minute or until heated through. Stir in lime juice and parsley or cilantro and remove from heat. Transfer vegetable mixture to a plate and keep warm.
	2. In the same skillet over medium heat, add eggs. Cook, stirring occasionally, until eggs are cooked through. Stir in vegetable mixture. Add cheese and cover skillet. Remove from heat and allow cheese to melt.
	3. Divide egg mixture among tortillas. Add salsa to taste and wrap tortillas around filling burrito-style. Serve immediately or allow to cool and wrap in plastic or foil to go.
Suggested Spice, Side or Condiment	Homemade salsa, Sriracha, Cholula,vegan ketchup

Meal # 6	"B.B.'s Cinnamon Roll French Toast"
Ingredients	Gluten-free cinnamon raisin bread, eggs, almond milk, vanilla coconut manna, raw honey, salt, cinnamon, pecans
Substitutions	Any gluten free bread, 100% wheat, or Ezekiel Bread
Shopping List	Gluten-free Cinnamon Raisin bread, eggs, almond milk, vanilla coconut manna, raw honey, salt, Cinnamon, pecans, Coconut Oil
Preparation	2 slices of gluten-free Cinnamon Raisin bread 1 whole egg Splash of almond milk Splash of vanilla 1 tbsp coconut manna 1 tbsp raw honey Pinch of salt 1-2 tbsp filtered water Cinnamon Chopped pecans

Cooking Instructions	Whisk eggs with almond milk and vanilla in a bowl.
	Dip each piece of bread in the egg mixture to coat. Let it soak in well so you don't have any eggs left over.
	Fry in coconut oil until golden brown on both sides.
	To make the glaze, combine coconut manna, raw honey and 1 tbsp water in a small saucepan on low heat and stir to combine.
	Add more water as needed to achieve a pourable "glaze" consistency.
Suggested Spice, Side or Condiment	Drizzle each slice with the honey-coconut glaze and sprinkle with chopped pecans. Add a sprinkle of cinnamon if desired. Real maple syrup 1 oz, butter 1 tablespoon

Meal # 7	"Ballin Bagel"
Ingredients	Whole Grain Bagel and Butter
Substitutions	*Pumpernickel, Rye Bagel, Gluten Free Bagel, Avocado or Hummus*
Shopping List	Go to nearest bagel store, treat yourself. There's no substitute for a fresh bagel. If you're not in NY, we are sorry for you. Find the closest thing to it or order a dozen bagels from NY to get you through the Diet plan.
Suggestions	Enjoy it!
Preparation	1 Bagel, Up to 2 tablespoons of butter
Cooking Instructions	Order a toasted bagel with plenty of butter or toast a bagel and smother it with butter.
Suggested Spice, Side or Condiment	Add 4 oz lox, chopped chives, Chopped red onions

Meal # 8	"Mr. Fancy Pants Quiche"
Ingredients	Brown Rice, Cheddar Cheese, Parmesan Cheese, Eggs, Broccoli, Nutmeg, Scallions
Substitutions	*Spinach*
Shopping List	Brown Rice, Cheddar Cheese, Parmesan Cheese, Eggs, Broccoli, Nutmeg, Scallions, Pie Crust, Salt, pepper
Suggestions	Bake ahead of time and let stand. Reheat, Use as more than one meal.
Preparation	Brown Rice (cooked), 2 cup • Egg, fresh, 5 large • Soy Milk, 1 cup • Broccoli, cooked, 2 cup, chopped • Cheddar Cheese, 1.25 cup, shredded Nutmeg, ground, .25 tsp
Cooking Instructions	Mix the rice, finely grated cheese and one egg in a bowl. Press the rice mixture into a pie plate, about 1/4 inch thick. Bake in a preheated 450 degree F oven until the edges and bottom just start turning golden brown, about 5 to 7 minutes. Mix the remaining eggs, milk, broccoli, sharp cheddar cheese and green onions in a bowl and season

	with salt and pepper. Pour the egg mixture into the pie crust.
	Bake in a preheated 375 degree F oven until golden brown and set in the center, about 30 to 35 minutes
	Serving Size: makes 6 servings
Suggested Spice, Side or Condiment	Fresh Salsa, Sriracha, Cholula

Meal # 9	"Baby Veggie Frittatas"
Ingredients	Red bell pepper, Yellow bell pepper, diced, zucchini, onion, Parmesan cheese, eggs.
Substitutions	*Broccoli, Asparagus*
Shopping List	Red bell pepper, Yellow bell pepper, Yellow and Green zucchini squash, onion, Parmesan cheese, Eggs,. Chives, Olive Oil
Suggestions	Frittatas can be tricky and turn out very easily as burned scrambled eggs.
Preparation	1 red bell pepper, diced

	1 yellow bell pepper, diced
	1 zucchini, diced
	1 small onion, diced
	1 cup Parmesan cheese
	8-10 eggs, beaten together
	2 tbsp chives
	salt and pepper to taste
	olive oil for drizzling
Cooking Instructions	Preheat oven to 350 degrees. In a large 10 inch skillet heat the olive oil over medium high heat. Saute the diced zucchini, onion and red and yellow bell peppers for about 5 minutes until they are slightly soft. Season with salt and pepper. Add the sauteed vegetables to individual muffin molds.
	1. In another bowl, whisk together 8 eggs and season with salt and pepper and add the chopped chives. Fill the remaining area in the muffin tin with the egg and stir the

	ingredients together. Sprinkle the top with the Parmesan cheese. Bake in the oven for 10-12 minutes until the eggs are completely set. Serve warm or cold.
Suggested Spice, Side or Condiment	Chives, Sriracha, Vegan Ketchup, Homemade Salsa

Meal # 10	"Bible Toast"
Ingredients	Ezekiel Toast, Bananas, and Natural Peanut Butter
Substitutions	*Blueberries, Strawberries, Almond Butter*
Shopping List	Ezekiel Toast, Bananas, and Natural Peanut Butter
Suggestions	This is a great energy breakfast and very filling!
Preparation	Prepare two slices of ezekiel bread, slice 1 banana into half inch discs, prepare 2 oz natural peanut butter.
Cooking Instructions	Toast 2 pieces of ezekiel bread, smother each side with natural peanut butter (2 oz), Place sliced bananas on each slice of toast, plate and eat.
Suggested Spice, Side or Condiment	Local Honey

Meal # 11	"Squash Latkes and Scrambled Eggs"
Ingredients	1 small spaghetti squash
	1/4 cup thinly sliced green onions
	1/4 cup finely chopped parsley
	5 sage leaves, finely chopped
	2 garlic cloves, minced
	1 large egg
	1/4 cup Pecorino Romano, grated
	1/4 cup chickpea flour
	1 teaspoon salt
	1/2 teaspoon freshly ground black pepper
	Peanut oil for frying
Substitutions	*Any other squash or serve with falafels*
Shopping List	Eggs, butter, spaghetti squash,romano cheese,parsley, sage, garlic, peanut oil
Suggestions	Pre make latkes and refrigerate before frying. Will hold well for up to 2 days in the fridge.

Preparation	Cut squash in half, scrape seeds, mince garlic, chop parsley, slice onions thin.
Cooking Instructions	Preheat oven to 400°F. Cut the squash in half lengthwise and scoop out the seeds. Lightly drizzle the flesh with olive oil and season with salt and pepper. Roast in the oven, cut-side up for about 40-50 minutes or until tender. Allow squash to cool slightly, then use a fork to shred the squash into strands. Transfer your squash "noodles" to a strainer to drain any excess liquid. In a large bowl, combine the sliced green onions, chopped parsley, chopped sage leaves, and minced garlic. Once the spaghetti strands have drained of excess liquid, add them to the bowl with the herbs and toss to coat. Fold in the egg, Pecorino Romano, chickpea flour, salt, and pepper. Toss all ingredients together until the mixture is well combined. Using a soup spoon, scoop a generous amount of the squash mixture into your hands and form into patties, one by one, and lightly flatten. Make sure you shape all of

	your patties before heating the oil. Heat one tablespoon of peanut oil in a large pan. Once the oil is hot (you can test by adding a strand of squash — if it sizzles, you're ready to go), add the patties, making sure not to overcrowd the pan. Depending on the pan size, you should be able to fry about 4 to 5 latkes at a time. Fry for about 2 minutes, or until golden brown and crispy. Flip the latkes and fry for another 2 minutes on the other side. Transfer the cooked latkes onto a paper towel–lined plate. Repeat with the rest of the mixture and additional peanut oil.
	Serving size 2 latkes accompanied by 2 scrambled eggs drizzled with butter.
Suggested Spice, Side or Condiment	Fresh salsa, tahini, Sriracha, Cholula, vegan ketchup

Meal # 12	"Amy's Omelette"
Ingredients	Egg Whites, broccoli, cheddar, butter
Substitutions	*Any cruciferous vegetable or cheese*
Shopping List	Eggs or egg whites, broccoli, butter, shredded cheddar
Suggestions	Add into a gluten free whole wheat wrap
Preparation	Lightly scramble three egg whites and chop broccoli into small chunks shred 2 oz cheddar.
Cooking Instructions	Add butter to hot saute pan Coat pan with butter as it melts Add broccoli and let cook for 3-5 minutes (smaller pieces will cook faster) Add egg whites Cook thoroughly and flip Add cheese to cooked side Fold and plate omelette
Suggested Spice, Side or Condiment	Vegan ketchup, fresh salsa, Sriracha, Cholula

Meal # 13	"Irish Farmer Breakfast"
Ingredients	Eggs, brown bread or grain bread, mushrooms, tomatoes, vegan bacon
Substitutions	*Any vegetables*
Shopping List	Eggs, brown bread or grain bread, mushrooms, tomatoes, vegan bacon, butter
Suggestions	Cook vegetables first
Preparation	Slice 2 pieces of bread Slice mushrooms Slice ½ tomato Prepare 2 pieces vegan bacon Prepare 1 tablespoon Butter
Cooking Instructions	In a non-stick pan saute mushrooms and tomatoes in butter and keep warm At the same time: Cook eggs "over hard" Fry 2 pieces of vegan bacon Toast 2 pieces whole grain bread Serve all on one plate
Suggested Spice, Side or Condiment	Sriracha, fresh salsa, butter, salt and pepper

Meal # 14	"Pedro's Toast"
Ingredients	Whole grain bread, refried beans, avocado
Substitutions	*Guacamole, hummus*
Shopping List	Whole grain bread, refried beans, avocado
Suggestions	This is a great energy packed breakfast. Enjoy it.
Preparation	2 Slices whole grain bread Portion 4 oz refried beans I whole avocado sliced
Cooking Instructions	Toast the bread, Spread refried beans on each slice, Layer avocado slices on top of refried beans
Suggested Spice, Side or Condiment	Sprinkle 2 oz shredded cheddar

LUNCH

Meal # 15	"The Bomb" Veggie Burger
Ingredients	<ul><li>Peanut oil</li><li>½ pound porcini mushrooms, trimmed and sliced</li><li>¾ teaspoon kosher salt,</li><li>Black pepper, as needed</li><li>1 (15-ounce) can kidney beans, drained</li><li>1 medium beet, peeled and coarsely grated (3/4 cup)</li><li>¾ cup cashews</li><li>⅓ cup panko bread crumbs</li><li>2 ounces queso blanco, crumbled or grated (about 1/2 cup)</li><li>2 large Organic eggs</li><li>2 tablespoons vegan mayonnaise</li><li>2 scallions, finely chopped</li><li>3 garlic cloves, finely chopped</li><li>¾ teaspoon paprika</li><li>4 ounces tempeh, crumbled</li><li>½ cup cooked brown rice</li><li>4 ounces extra-firm tofu, drained</li></ul>
Substitutions	*Dr. Praeger's Frozen Veggie Burger*

Shopping List	Tofu, Mushrooms, Kosher Salt, garlic, Cashews, Panko Breadcrumbs, Scallions, Paprika, Tempeh, Brown Rice, Beet, Kidney Beans, Organic Eggs, Queso Blanco.
Suggestions	Add a slice of cheese of your choice.
Preparation	Heat oven to 425 degrees. Slice tofu into 1/4-inch-thick slabs and pat dry with paper towels. Arrange tofu on one half of a rimmed baking sheet; brush both sides with oil. Spread mushrooms on the other half of the baking sheet; toss with 2 tablespoons oil and salt and pepper. On a second rimmed baking sheet, toss beans and grated beet with 1 tablespoon oil and salt and pepper, then spread the mixture into one layer. Transfer both baking sheets to the oven. Roast bean-beet mixture, tossing occasionally, until beans begin to split and beets are tender and golden, about 15 minutes. Roast

mushrooms and tofu until golden and most of the liquid has evaporated, about 25 minutes. Let everything cool.

Place nuts in a food processor and pulse until coarsely ground. Add cooled bean-beet mixture, mushrooms, tofu, panko, cheese, eggs, mayonnaise, scallion, garlic, pimentón and 3/4 teaspoon salt. Pulse until ingredients are just combined. Pulse in tempeh and rice but do not over process. You want small chunks, not a smooth mixture. Scrape mixture into a bowl and chill at least 2 hours or up to 5 days (you can also freeze the burger mix).

When you are ready to make the burgers, divide mixture into 6 equal portions and form each portion into a patty about 1 inch thick. Return to the fridge until just before grilling.

	They grill better when they start out cold.
Cooking Instructions	Heat the grill or Skillet

Cook the burgers over a low fire until they are charred on both sides and firm when you press on them, 4 to 6 minutes per side. If they start to burn before they firm up, move them to the sides of the grill to finish cooking over indirect heat. Alternatively, you can cook these on a grill pan or skillet over low heat. |
| Suggested Spice, Side or Condiment | Vegan ketchup, vegan BBQ sauce, sliced tomato, lettuce, red onion, baked french fries |

Meal # 16	"The Dark Side" Veggie Burger
Ingredients	Black Beans, thai chili sauce, onion, green pepper, garlic, chili powder, cumin, whole grain bun, cheddar cheese
Substitutions	*Red or Yellow Peppers*
Shopping List	Black Beans, thai chili sauce, onion, green pepper, garlic, chili powder, cumin, whole grain bun, cheddar cheese, eggs
Suggestions	These are delicious. You'll crush it!
Preparation	1 tablespoon cumin 1 teaspoon Thai chili sauce or cholula hot sauce 1/2 cup bread crumbs 1 (16 ounce) can black beans, drained and rinsed 1/2 green bell pepper, cut into 2 inch pieces 1/2 onion, cut into wedges

	3 cloves garlic, peeled
	1 Organic egg
	1 tablespoon chili powder
	In a medium bowl, mash black beans with a fork until thick and pasty.
	In a food processor, finely chop bell pepper, onion, and garlic. Then stir into mashed beans.
	In a small bowl, stir together egg, chili powder, cumin, and chili sauce.
	Stir the egg mixture into the mashed beans. Mix in bread crumbs until the mixture is sticky and holds together. Divide mixture into four patties.
Cooking Instructions	If grilling, preheat an outdoor grill for high heat, and lightly oil a sheet of aluminum foil. If baking, preheat oven to 375 degrees F (190 degrees C), and lightly oil a baking sheet.If

	grilling, place patties on foil, and grill about 8 minutes on each side. If baking, place patties on a baking sheet, and bake about 10 minutes on each side.
Suggested Spice, Side or Condiment	Vegan ketchup, vegan BBQ sauce, sliced tomato, lettuce, red onion, baked french fries

Meal # 17	"Charlie the Tuna" Salad
Ingredients	Fresh tuna, red onion, creole mustard, vegan mayo, celery
Substitutions	*Swordfish, Mako Shark*
Shopping List	8 oz Fresh tuna steak, red onion, creole mustard, vegan mayo, celery
Suggestions	Try recipe with smoked fish
Preparation	8 oz tuna steak ¼ cup diced red onions 2 oz vegan mayo 2 oz creole mustard ¼ cup diced celery Salt and pepper

Cooking Instructions	In a medium saute pan heat peanut oil and cook tuna steak approximately 3-5 minutes on both sides. Tuna should be cooked through completely. Once tuna is cooked remove from pan and break apart. Fish should flake away easily. Place in refrigerator and let chill. Once cold, mix all ingredients in a bowl. Use a fork.
Suggested Spice, Side or Condiment	Serve Over lettuce or on a Whole Grain Roll or Whole Grain Wrap

Meal # 18	**"Over the Wall" Guacamole and Chips**
Ingredients	Avocado, cilantro, tomato, red onion, garlic, olive oil, black bean chips
Substitutions	*Any Non-Flour Baked Chip, Toast Points or Fresh Veggies*
Shopping List	Avocado, cilantro, tomato, red onion, garlic, olive oil, black bean chips
Preparation	1 avocado 1 tablespoons minced onion 1 tablespoons lime juice, or more to taste ¼ teaspoon sea salt, or more to taste 2 oz cilantro chopped fine 1 Clove garlic minced

	1 Fresh tomatoes chopped 6 oz black bean chips
Cooking Instructions	Combine the onion, lime juice and salt in a medium bowl. Peel and pit the avocados and add to the bowl. Mash with potato masher until combined. Taste and add more lime juice and salt if needed. Serve with Chips
Suggested Spice, Side or Condiment	Fresh salsa

Meal # 19	"Miami Grilled Cheese" With Tomato and Avocado
Ingredients	Whole grain bread, gruyere or swiss, cheddar, tomato, avocado, hummus, butter, vegan mayo
Substitutions	*Fresh guacamole*
Shopping List	Whole grain bread, gruyere or swiss, cheddar, tomato, avocado, hummus, butter, vegan mayo
Preparation	2 slices Whole grain bread Tablespoon Butter, 2 slices sharp cheddar cheese, 2 slices gruyere, 1 avocado sliced, vegan mayo, 2 slices tomato
Cooking Instructions	Place alternating cheese slices on both halves of bread covered with layer of hummus, 2 slices tomato on one side, place avocado slices on

	top of tomato, now place sandwich together and press firmly. Prepare hot non-stick pan. Spread vegan mayo on outside layer of bread and place sandwich mayo side down in hot pan. While sandwich is in pan spread mayo on the dry side of bread. Flip once and use a burger press or some weighted object to press the sandwich down. 3-5 minutes on each side
Suggested Spice, Side or Condiment	Tahini sauce, or chipotle spiced vegan mayo

Meal # 20	"Southwest Black Bean Soup"
Ingredients	Black beans, cheddar cheese, Vegan Sour Cream
Substitutions	*Fat free sour Cream, and cheese*
Suggestions	This is a great, easy to make filling meal
Cooking Instructions	Heat black bean soup, sprinkle 2 oz cheddar cheese and tablespoon vegan sour cream
Suggested Spice, Side or Condiment	Chili Powder

Meal # 21	"The Grizzly" Broiled Salmon with Broccoli Rabe
Ingredients	8 oz Wild Salmon, Broccoli Rabe, Garlic
Substitutions	*Any Green Cruciferous Vegetable, Cod or Halibut*
Shopping List	Wild Salmon, Fresh Broccoli Rabe, Peanut Oil, Garlic
Suggestions	Broccoli is a good substitute
Preparation	Wash Broccoli rabe, Cut off long stalks
Cooking Instructions	Spray baking dish with cooking spray and place salmon on dish. Add a ¼ cup of water to baking dish and place in preheated 375 degree oven. Bring a large pot of salted water to boil. Set up a bowl of well salted ice

	water. Drop the broccoli rabe into the boiling water and cook for 1 minute. Remove from the boiling water and plunge immediately into the ice water. Once cool remove from the ice water and let dry. It can be used right away or held for future use.
	Coat a large saute pan with peanut oil. Add the smashed garlic and crushed red pepper and bring to medium heat. Once the garlic is brown and aromatic, remove it from the pan and discard. It has fulfilled its garlic destiny. Add the broccoli rabe and toss around in the oil to heat up and season. Remember the broccoli is already cooked. Add more oil, if needed and season with salt if needed
Suggested Spice, Side or Condiment	Wasabi Spiced Vegan Mayo

Meal # 22	"The Border Patrol" Meatless Burrito
Ingredients	**1 cup** Brown Rice, 1 can black beans, 4 oz shredded jack cheese, 2 oz Vegan sour cream, 4 oz guacamole, 1 Large Whole wheat or Whole Grain Tortilla
Substitutions	*Grilled Vegetables*
Shopping List	Brown Rice, black beans, shredded jack cheese, Vegan sour cream, guacamole, Whole wheat or Whole Grain Tortilla
Suggestions	Many options for substitutions here. Just follow the rules and portion sizes.

Preparation	Cook brown rice as per package directions Warm black beans on stove top and drain Spread cheese followed by rice, drained black, guacamole, and sour cream. Fold and wrap burrito tightly, cut in half and plate
Suggested Spice, Side or Condiment	Sriracha, Cholula, Green Chile Sauce

Meal # 23 (for 2 people)	"Old School Wrap" Grilled Vegetable Wrap
Ingredients	1 Red pepper, 1 Red onion, 1 yellow and 1 green squash, 6 Stalks Asparagus, 4 oz feta cheese, 2 whole grain wraps or pitas.
Substitutions	*Gorgonzola, Goat cheese, And vegetables*
Shopping List	Red pepper, onion, yellow and green squash, Asparagus, feta cheese, a whole grain wrap or pita, Vegan Grill Spray, Garlic Powder, Balsamic Vinegar, Peanut Oil
Suggestions	Dry the vegetables on paper towel to soak up moisture. They'll make a mess of your wrap.
Preparation	Cut all vegetables julienne style

Cooking Instructions	If grilling, spray grill and place vegetables on grill facing opposite direction. Cook until soft.
	If cooking in oven, place on ventilated baking rack in preheated 375 degree oven. Place in large bowl and toss with salt and pepper and a ¼ cup of balsamic vinegar. Drain on paper towels. Place in wrap with feta cheese touching wrap side.
Suggested Spice, Side or Condiment	Small salad

Meal # 24	"Upper East Side" Garden Reuben
Ingredients	2 slices Fresh 100% Rye Bread, 1 slice Swiss or gruyere Cheese, ¼ cup sauerkraut, 1 "the bomb" or "dark side" veggie burger, butter, vegan thousand island dressing
Substitutions	*lentil pattie, falafel patty.*
Shopping List	100% Rye Bread, Swiss or Gruyere, Sauerkraut, List from veggie burger
Suggestions/Comments	Nothing but pure love here. You'll feel like you're cheating. Pure awesomeness!
Preparation	Make veggie burger patty as per "The bomb" or the "Dark Side' recipe. ¼ cup sauerkraut 1 oz vegan thousand island 1 slice cheese 1 Tablespoon butter

Cooking Instructions	Preheat a large skillet or griddle on medium heat for sandwich
	Heat veggie burgers and sauerkraut in separate pan or bake in the oven at 375 for 15 minutes
	Lightly butter one side of both bread slices. Spread non-buttered sides with Thousand Island dressing.Add veggie burger, sauerkraut and cheese. Press sides together to make sandwich.
	Grill sandwich until both sides are golden brown, about 15 minutes per side. Serve hot.
Suggested Spice, Side or Condiment	Serve with extra Vegan Thousand Island for dipping

Meal # 25	"The Big House" Falafel with Broccoli Slaw and Tahini in Pita
Ingredients	<ul><li>1 cups Broccoli Cole Slaw</li><li>1/4 cup vinaigrette</li><li>1/4 cup Red onion, thinly sliced</li><li>6 Falafels</li><li>1/4 cup Hummus</li><li>1 Pocket-style pitas, halved and split open</li><li>1/4 cup Tahini sauce</li></ul>
Substitutions	*Veggie burgers, Lentil patties*
Shopping List	Broccoli Cole Slaw, Sugar Free Vinaigrette, Red onion, Falafel Powder, Chickpeas or Hummus, Pocket-style whole wheat or whole grain pitas,Tahini sauce

Suggestions	You can save some steps by purchasing premade broccoli slaw, hummus, and tahini. Be aware of the sugar content.
Preparation	Toss together broccoli coleslaw, vinaigrette and red onion; set aside. Meanwhile, prepare falafels according to package directions. Spread hummus on the inside of each pita half; stuff with Broccoli Cole Slaw and warm falafels. Drizzle with tahini sauce. Serve immediately with remaining cole slaw on the side.
Cooking Instructions	Fry: Mix water and **falafel** mix; let stand 15 minutes. Pour 1 inch peanut oil into a deep pan; heat oil to 350-375°F. Make small balls and

	fry until brown and crisp; drain on paper towels.
	Bake: Grease a large rimmed baking sheet with 2 tablespoons of oil. Roll the bean mixture into 20 balls, about 1½ inches each, then flatten them into thick patties. Put the **falafel** on the prepared pan and brush the tops with the remaining 2 tablespoons oil. **Bake** until golden all over, 10 to 15 minutes on each side.
Suggested Spice, Side or Condiment	Tahini

Meal # 26	"Montauk Fish Burger"
Ingredients	Fresh tuna steaks,carrots, onions, chives,eggs,panko bread crumbs, vegan mayo,garlic salt, pepper, olive oil
Substitutions	*Salmon burger, fish cake, crab cake.*
Shopping List	8 oz fresh Tuna Steak, Fresh parsley, carrot, onion, chives,eggs,panko bread crumbs, vegan mayo,garlic salt, pepper, olive oil
Suggestions	
Preparation	<ul><li>8oz fresh tuna steaks, minced</li><li>1 carrot, grated</li><li>¼ cup chopped parsley</li><li>1/2 cup onion, chopped</li><li>1/2 cup chopped fresh chives</li><li>2 eggs</li><li>1/3 cup panko crumbs or</li></ul>

	breadcrumbs
	<ul><li>1 tablespoon mayonnaise</li><li>garlic salt to taste</li><li>freshly ground black pepper to taste</li></ul>
Cooking Instructions	In a large bowl, mix together tuna, carrots, onions, chives, eggs, panko crumbs, and mayonnaise. Season with garlic salt and black pepper. Form into patties. 1. Heat the oil in a skillet over medium heat. Arrange patties in the pan (only as many as will fit easily in the pan). Cook, uncovered, 10 minutes per side, or until golden brown.
Suggested Spice, Side or Condiment	Serve on Whole Grain Bun with Lettuce and Tomato, Vegan Tartar

Meal # 27	"RockStar Salad" Gorgonzola and Walnut Salad
Ingredients	4 oz Mesclun Greens 2 oz Gorgonzola Cheese 1 Pear 2oz Walnuts 2oz Fresh Cranberries 4 oz Grape Tomatoes 2 oz Red Onions
Substitutions	*Add 4 Shrimp, Sliced whole avocado for protein*
Shopping List	Mesclun Greens, Gorgonzola Cheese, Pears, Walnuts, Fresh Cranberries, Grape Tomatoes, Red Onions, Sugar free dressing
Suggestions	A great base for many other dishes. You can add veggie burger, falafel, shrimp. Count as a your big meal if doing this!

Preparation	Greens first, Layer on your ingredients
Suggested Spice, Side or Condiment	Sugar free dressing

Meal # 28	"Renaissance Caesar"
Ingredients	4 oz Vegan caesar dressing 4 oz Romaine Lettuce 2 oz Shaved Parm 2 oz Toasted Pine Nuts 2 oz Whole Grain Croutons
Shopping List	Vegan caesar dressing Romaine Lettuce Shaved Parm Toasted Pine Nuts Whole Grain Croutons
Preparation	Chop romaine into 2 inch squares and place in bowl Pour in dressing and hand mix until the lettuce is coated with dressing. Top with pine nuts, shaved parm, and croutons
Suggested Spice, Side or Condiment	Fresh pepper

Meal # 29	"Popeye's Mistress" Spinach Salad with Goat Cheese and Vegan Bacon Bits
Ingredients	4 oz Spinach salad 2 oz Goat Cheese 4 oz Vegan Bacon 4 oz Sugar free dressing
Substitutions	*Turkey bacon bits*
Shopping List	Baby Spinach, Goat Cheese crumbles, Vegan Bacon, Sugar free dressing
Suggestions	You can drizzle hot bacon drippings over salad for added flavor
Preparation	Place spinach in bowl, Top with bacon bits first and then goat cheese. top with dressing and bacon drippings. Serve immediately.

Meal # 30	"The Bounty" Garden Salad
Ingredients	4 oz romaine or Iceberg 2 oz shredded carrot 6 Grape tomatoes 2 radishes sliced 2 oz Sliced red onion 2 oz Roasted Red Peppers Sugar free dressing
Substitutions	
Shopping List	Romaine or Iceberg lettuce, carrots, Grape tomatoes, Radishes, Red Onion, Roasted Red Peppers
Suggestions	Substitute any vegetables. Keep portions the same just substitute as to your preference.
Preparation	No rules. Enjoy!
Suggested Spice, Side or Condiment	Vegan dressing

DINNER

Dinner is considered your "big" meal for the day but feel free to have your big meal for lunch and substitute a lunch item or even a breakfast item for dinner.

Meal # 31	"The Beach" Seafood Pasta
Ingredients	4 Clams, 4 Shrimp, 12 Mussels, 1/4 Lb. Gluten Free or Whole Wheat Pasta, 2 oz Olive Oil, 1 clove garlic, 4 oz White Wine, 2 oz Fresh Parsley, 2 Shallots, 2 oz Fresh Parmesan
Substitutions	*Any seafood, match the portions*
Shopping List	Littleneck clams, 16-20 size shrimp,mussels, gluten free or whole wheat pasta, olive oil, garlic, white wine - chardonnay or chablis, parsley, shallots, pecorino romano cheese
Preparation	Clean shrimp, scrub mussels, wash clams in fresh water.

	Chop parsley fine Mince garlic Slice shallots thin
Cooking Instructions	Cook pasta al dente In separate large saute pan heat olive oil Add clams, parsley, shallots, and garlic. Simmer for 3 minutes. Add white wine and cover until clams begin to open. Add mussels and shrimp. As soon as and mussels are open and shrimp are red add cooked pasta. Toss and serve immediately. Sprinkle romano cheese
Suggested Spice, Side or Condiment	Whole grain roll

Meal # 32	"The Flatty" Broiled Fish with Baked Sweet Potato and Asparagus
Ingredients	8oz flounder, 1 sweet potato, 4 oz asparagus, 1 lemon, almonds, tablespoon butter, 2 oz white wine
Substitutions	*Halibut, Fluke, Sole*
Shopping List	8 oz fresh flounder filet, sweet potatoes, asparagus, butter, shaved almonds
Preparation	Chop 1 inch of butt ends of asparagus Cut lemon into wedges Wash sweet potato
Cooking Instructions	Bake sweet potato for 45 minutes at 400 Cook asparagus in pan with 1 cup water and a pinch of salt. Cook until soft or to desired firmness.

	Flat fish cooks very quickly. You can either saute for 3 minutes on each side or bake for 7-10 minutes at 400. In a saute pan; heat olive oil, add almonds, butter and white wine, squeeze 3 wedges of lemon juice into pan. Cook for 2 minutes or until almonds are starting to brown. Remove from heat and pour directly over fish. Plate with hot sweet potato and asparagus.
Suggested Spice, Side or Condiment	A little extra butter for sweet potato

Meal # 33	"Wild and Shrimpy" Shrimp Scampi with brown rice and sauteed spinach.
Ingredients	6 shrimp, 4 oz spinach, 1 cup of brown rice, 2 cloves garlic,1 tablespoon butter, 4oz white wine, 1 oz peanut oil
Substitutions	Sea Scallops
Shopping List	16-20 size shrimp, baby spinach, brown rice, garlic, butter, white wine - chardonnay or chablis
Cooking Instructions	In a hot medium saute pan add peanut oil and shrimp. As soon as shrimp begin to turn red add garlic and butter. Boil rice as per package directions.

	As soon as the butter is melted add white wine and let simmer for 3 minutes.
	In separate pan saute spinach with 1 tablespoon butter and remaining garlic until wilted
	Plate spinach and rice. Place shrimp over rice and drizzle juice from shrimp pan over shrimp and rice.
Suggested Spice, Side or Condiment	Cholula, Lemon

Meal # 34	"Wednesday Night Meeting"
	Vegetable Lasagna
Ingredients	1 1/2 quarts spaghetti sauce (your favorite homemade or jar spaghetti sauce) 1/2 cup grated carrot 1/2 teaspoon oregano 6 cooked lasagna noodles 1 (16 ounce) containers ricotta cheese 1 bag fresh baby spinach, thawed and well drained 2 eggs 1 1/2 cups thinly sliced yellow and green squash 1 cup sliced portobello 3 cups shredded part-skim mozzarella cheese 1/2 cup grated parmesan cheese

Substitutions	
Shopping List	Pasta sauce, Carrots, oregano, gluten-free lasagna noodles, ricotta cheese, baby spinach, onions, green and yellow squash
Suggestions	
Preparation	○ 1. Mix carrots, oregano, and spaghetti sauce together. 2. Mix Ricotta, spinach, and eggs together in separate bowl. 3. Spread ½ cup spaghetti sauce in bottom of 9 x 13 inch baking dish. 4. Layer 3 lasagna noodles, ½ remaining sauce, ½ Ricotta mixture, ½ sliced zucchini, ½ sliced mushrooms, ½ Mozzarella, and ½ Parmesan. 5. Repeat layers with remaining ingredients.
Cooking Instructions	Bake in a 350 degree oven for about 45-60 minutes.

Suggested Spice, Side or Condiment	Side Salad or Broccoli Rabe and Whole Grain Roll

Meal # 35	"Island Dream" Lentil Patties with Lettuce and Tahini Sauce
Ingredients	1½ cups red lentils 3 cups water 1 onion, finely diced 2 cloves garlic, finely minced 2 tsp garam masala 1 tsp cumin seed 2 eggs ½ cup whole wheat flour 1 tsp salt 1 tsp fresh ground black pepper ¼ cup finely chopped cilantro Peanut Oil
Shopping List	Red lentils, onion, garlic, garam masala, cumin seed, organic eggs, whole wheat flour, cilantro, peanut oil
Preparation	In a large saucepan, bring lentils and water to boil. Reduce the heat to low and simmer for 10 minutes,

	or until the lentils are very soft. Drain the lentils well.
	Meanwhile, in a large heavy-bottomed skillet, saute the onion in olive oil for 5-7 minutes, or until onion is soft and golden-brown. Add garlic, cumin seed and garam masala, and continue cooking for 2 minutes or until garlic is soft and spices are fragrant. Remove from heat.
	In a large mixing bowl, combine the cooked lentils, sauteed onions, eggs, flour, salt, pepper and cilantro.
Cooking Instructions	In a large heavy-bottomed skillet, heat 2 tbsp canola oil over medium-high heat. Working in

	batches, use a ¼ cup measure to drop batter into the hot oil and flatten out into ¾" thick patties using a spatula. Fry the patties for 5 minutes per side or until golden-brown and crisp, adding more oil to the pan as necessary. Serve warm or at room temperature
Suggested Spice, Side or Condiment	Side Salad and Tahini Sauce

Meal # 36	"The Sizzling Platter" Skillet Cooked Shrimp Fajitas with Peppers and Zucchini
Ingredients	6 medium shrimp, peeled and deveined 1/4 teaspoon salt 1/4 teaspoon ground cumin 1/4 teaspoon pure chile powder 1/4 teaspoon chopped oregano 1/4 teaspoon garlic powder Juice of ½ lime 1 Large Whole Wheat or Whole Grain Tortilla 1/2 tablespoons vegetable oil ½ green onion, cut into quarters

	1 green bell peppers, cut into 1/3 inch strips ½ cup Vegan sour cream 1 Teaspoon chopped fresh cilantro ¼ minced red onion
Substitutions	*Sea scallops*
Shopping List	6 medium shrimp, peeled and deveined, salt ground cumin Chile powder,oregano, garlic powder, lime, Whole Wheat or Whole Grain Tortillas, Peanut oil,onion, green bell pepper, Vegan sour cream, fresh cilantro, red onion
Suggestions	Use a cast iron skillet. Great cooking tool!
Preparation	Add shrimp, salt, cumin, chile powder, oregano, garlic, lime juice

	to a large bowl or heavy duty zip-top plastic bag.
	Toss until spices are distributed and shrimp is well coated.
	Let marinate for 10 minutes.
Cooking Instructions	Heat the oil in a large skillet (cast-iron is best).
	Add green onions and peppers; cook and stir occasionally for 2 minutes or until slightly softened.
	Add shrimp and marinade; cook and stir constantly for about 3 minutes or until the shrimp are pink.
	Spoon shrimp and vegetables into warmed tortillas; garnish with sour cream, cilantro and onion if desired.Fold up and eat.

Suggested Spice, Side or Condiment	Cholula, Green Chile

Meal # **37**	**"Summer Lovin"** **Marinated Seafood Salad with Chickpeas and Parmesan**
Ingredients	1 cups water 1/4 cup white wine vinegar 1/2 teaspoon kosher salt 6 large shrimp (16-20 size shrimp), peeled and deveined ¼ pound sea scallops (10 to 12 size) 1/2 pound fresh mussels in the shell, scrubbed and beards removed 1/4 cup olive oil 1/4 teaspoon whole fresh thyme leaves 1/2 teaspoon minced fresh garlic 1/2 lemon, zested Juice of half a lemon ½ teaspoon Dijon mustard

	½ tablespoons Champagne or white wine vinegar ½ teaspoons kosher salt Pinch freshly ground black pepper ¼ cup diced celery 1 tablespoons chopped fresh parsley leaves Thinly sliced lemon, for garnish ½ cup chickpeas
Substitutions	*Squid rings and tentacles*
Shopping List	white wine vinegar, kosher salt, 6 large shrimp (16-20 size shrimp), peeled and deveined, ¼ pound sea scallops (10 to 12 size), 1/2 pound fresh mussels in the shell, scrubbed and beards removed, olive oil, fresh thyme leaves, fresh garlic, lemon,, Dijon mustard, Champagne or white wine vinegar, black pepper, diced celery, fresh parsley, chickpeas
Cooking Instructions	To cook the seafood, combine 8 cups of water with the white wine

vinegar and salt in a large saucepan and bring to a boil. Add shrimp and cook for 2 minutes. Remove with a slotted spoon. Bring water back to a boil and cook the scallops for 4 to 5 minutes, until cooked through. Drain.

Bring 1/2 cup of water to boil in the same saucepan and toss in the mussels. Return to boil, cover, and steam for 3 to 5 minutes, until they're all opened. (Discard any that remain unopened after 5 minutes.) Drain. Remove the mussels from the shells and discard the shells. Drain all the cooked seafood and place it in a large bowl.

To make the sauce, heat the olive oil in a medium saute pan and add the thyme, garlic, and lemon zest. Cook over low heat for 1 minute. Off the heat, add the lemon juice, mustard, vinegar, salt, and pepper.

	Pour the hot vinaigrette over the seafood. Add the celery and parsley and toss well. This salad can be served immediately, but it is best when allowed to sit, refrigerated, for 1 to 2 hours. Sprinkle with salt and toss with sliced lemon.
Suggested Spice, Side or Condiment	Crusty Whole Grain Roll

Meal # 38	"Greek Goddess" Penne with Broccoli Rabe and Feta
Ingredients	¼ lb Whole Wheat Penne, 6oz broccoli rabe, 4 oz feta, 2 oz olive oil, ½ tablespoon chopped parsley, Garlic
Substitutions	*Broccoli, String beans, Peas, Spinach, Vegetable based pasta*
Shopping List	Whole Wheat or Gluten Free Pasta, Broccoli, Feta Crumbles, Olive Oil, garlic
Suggestions	Can be eaten cold as well.
Preparation	Cut stalks off or broccoli rabe Chop Parsley Chop garlic
Cooking Instructions	Cook pasta al dente

Bring a large pot of salted water to boil. Set up a bowl of well salted ice water. Drop the broccoli rabe into the boiling water and cook for 1 minute. Remove from the boiling water and plunge immediately into the ice water. Once cool remove from the ice water and let dry. It can be used right away or held for future use.

Coat a large saute pan with peanut oil. Add the smashed garlic and crushed red pepper and bring to medium heat. Once the garlic is brown and aromatic, remove it from the pan and discard. It has fulfilled its garlic destiny. Add the broccoli rabe and toss around in the oil to heat up and season. Remember the broccoli is already cooked. Add more oil, if needed and season with salt if needed

	Add cooked pasta, Toss toss with broccoli rabe. Place in a bowl and top with feta crumbles and fresh parsley
Suggested Spice, Side or Condiment	Fresh Pecorino Romano Parmesan

Meal # 39	"The Affair" Pistachio Crusted Halibut In Almond Milk Beurre Blanc Sauce
Ingredients	8 oz halibut filet
	¼ cup pistachio
	¼ cup whole wheat bread crumb
	tablespoon butter
	juice of half a lemon
	salt and pepper to taste
	4 oz asparagus
	1/3 cup orange juice
	2 tablespoons finely chopped shallot
	1-1/2 teaspoons minced fresh ginger root
	1 small garlic clove, minced
	1 can (13.66 ounces) light coconut milk
	1 teaspoon sugar
	1/8 teaspoon salt
	Dash pepper

	1 tablespoon butter
Substitutions	*Blackfish, Striped Bass, Wahu*
Shopping List	8oz halibut filet, ¼ cup pistachio, ¼ cup whole wheat bread crumb, tablespoon butter, juice of half a lemon, salt and pepper to taste , 4 oz asparagus
Suggestions	
Preparation	In food processor: Mix pistachio, butter, bread crumbs, lemon, salt and pepper and mix until all ingredients hold together. Sauce: In a small saucepan, combine the orange juice, shallots, ginger and garlic. Bring to a boil over medium-high heat. Cook for 3 minutes. Stir in coconut milk, sugar, salt and pepper. Simmer,

	stirring occasionally until mixture is reduced by half, about 20 minutes. Remove from the heat and whisk in butter.
Cooking Instructions	Spoon or hand press pistachio mixture onto top of fish forming a layer of crust

Place non-stick baking pan or sprayed saute pan and bake for 12-15 minutes at 400 degrees

Cook asparagus in pan with ½ cup water and a pinch of salt. Cook to desired firmness |

Meal # 40	"The Flemish Cap" **Grilled Swordfish Piccata with Baby Spinach and Sweet potato frites**
Ingredients	Six 6- to 7-ounce skinless swordfish steaks • Salt and freshly ground black pepper • 6 thin slices of serrano ham or prosciutto • 1/2 cup all-purpose flour, plus more for dusting • 1/2 cup freshly grated Parmigiano-Reggiano cheese • 1 large egg, beaten • 1/2 cup milk • 2 tablespoons extra-virgin olive oil • 1 stick unsalted butter • 1/2 cup sliced almonds • 2 tablespoons freshly squeezed lemon juice • 2 tablespoons drained capers

	• 2 tablespoons chopped flat-leaf parsley • Sautéed kale, creamy polenta and lemon wedges, for serving
Substitutions	*Mako, Tuna*
Shopping List	• 6- to 7-ounce skinless swordfish steaks • Salt and freshly ground black pepper • all-purpose flour • ham or prosciutto • Parmigiano-Reggiano cheese • Eggs • Milk • Extra-virgin olive oil • Unsalted butter • Sliced almonds • lemons • Capers • Flat-leaf parsley • Kale • Polenta • Baby Spinach

	• Sweet Potatoes
Suggestions	Use freshest cuts of fish
Preparation and Cooking Instructions	1. Preheat the oven to 350°. Season the swordfish steaks with salt and black pepper and wrap a slice of ham around each steak. Lightly dust the swordfish all over with flour.
	2. In a pie plate, combine the 1/2 cup of flour with grated Parmigiano-Reggiano cheese. In another pie plate, whisk the beaten egg with the milk. Dip the swordfish steaks in the egg mixture, allowing the excess to drip off, then press the steaks into the flour mixture so that it adheres.

3. In a large ovenproof nonstick skillet, heat the olive oil until shimmering. Add the swordfish steaks and cook over moderately high heat until lightly browned, about 3 minutes. Flip the steaks over. Transfer the skillet to the oven and roast the swordfish for about 5 minutes, until cooked through.

4. Meanwhile, in a medium skillet, melt the butter. Add the sliced almonds and cook over moderate heat, stirring, until the almonds are toasted and the butter is lightly browned, about 4 minutes. Remove the sauce from the heat and add the lemon juice, capers and parsley. Transfer the

	swordfish steaks to plates and spoon the sauce on top..
Suggested Spice, Side or Condiment	Horseradish Sauce, Lemon, Pepper

Meal # 41	"Baby Mama's Pizza"
Ingredients	Pre made 8 inch whole wheat pizza crust or tandoori bread 1 cup Baby Spinach 2 plum Tomatoes ½ cup Mushrooms ½ cup Bell Pepper 4 oz Shredded mozzarella Tablespoon Olive oil 1 clove Garlic
Substitutions	*Any local vegetables*
Shopping List	Pre made 8 inch whole wheat pizza crust or tandoori bread Baby Spinach Tomatoes Mushrooms Peppers Shredded mozzarella, Olive oil Garlic
Suggestions	Gluten free crust is a big project but recipe is here. Tandoori bread

	makes a great crispy pizza. Check out our cauliflower pizza crust!
Preparation	Slice 2 plum tomatoes very thin Slice mushrooms Mince 1 clove garlic Julienne pepper
Cooking Instructions	Cover the inside of crust with lightly sauteed plum tomatoes, top with sauteed spinach and mushrooms, sprinkle mozzarella cheese, brush exposed crust with olive oil
Suggested Spice, Side or Condiment	Side Salad

Meal # 42	"The Fairfield" Grilled Cheese With Apple
Ingredients	2 pc Whole Grain Sliced Bread 3 Slices Gruyere Half Green Apple Sliced Thin Vegan Mayo
Substitutions	*Any cheese*
Shopping List	Whole grain bread Gruyere cheese Green apple Vegan Mayo
Suggestions	
Preparation	Place 2 slices of cheese on 1 slice bread Place 1 slice cheese and a layer of apple slices on other side Combine as sandwich Spread vegan mayo on outside of 1 slice bread and place in hot pan.

	As soon as sandwich is placed in pan spread mayo on other side Flip sandwich and cook until cheese is melted.
Suggested Spice, Side or Condiment	Broccoli Slaw and Black Bean Chips

Meal # 43 (4 Servings)	"Straight out of The Bronx" Eggplant Parmesan
Ingredients	1 large eggplant, peeled and cut into 1/3 inch slices 2 eggs, beaten 1 1/2 cups seasoned dry whole wheat bread crumbs 1/4 cup olive oil 3 cups spaghetti sauce 1/2 lb shredded mozzarella cheese 1/3 cup grated parmesan cheese
Substitutions	
Shopping List	Eggplant Organic Eggs Whole Wheat Bread Crumbs

	Olive Oil
	Ingredients for sauce if making from scratch
	Part Skim Mozzarella Cheese
	Pecorino Romano Grated Cheese
	Ingredients for sauce if making from scratch
Preparation	1. Arrange a layer of eggplant slices in a colander. Sprinkle generously with salt. Continue layering and salting all eggplant slices. Let stand 30 minutes. Rinse and pat dry. Dip each eggplant slice in beaten egg, and dredge with breadcrumbs.
	2. Heat oil in a heavy skillet. Over medium high heat fry eggplant in hot oil about 2 minutes per side until golden. Drain on absorbent

	paper.
	3. Preheat oven to temperature 350°F Arrange half the eggplant slices in the bottom of baking dish sprayed lightly with nonstick spray. Spread half the sauce over top. Sprinkle with half the mozzarella and half the Parmesan. Repeat layers.
	4. Bake 20-25 minutes or until mixture is bubbly.
Suggested Spice, Side or Condiment	Whole Grain Roll, Salad

Meal # 44 (4 servings) *This your entire dairy allotment for day! No cheese on this day*	"Gloucester Docks" **Corn and Clam Chowder with fresh corn bread.**
Ingredients	2 ears shucked fresh corn on the cob, or 1 ½ cups canned whole kernel corn • 20 littleneck clams, the smaller the better • ½ large carrot, • 1 Stalk celery • ½ Onion • 2 sprigs fresh thyme • ½ cups dry white wine • 3 cups canned chicken broth • 1.5 cups heavy cream • Salt to taste • Freshly ground pepper to taste • 1/2 tablespoons freshly squeezed lime juice • 1 tablespoons butter • ½ small hot red or green peppers, stems removed

	- 1/2 tablespoons olive oil - ¼ cup finely chopped fresh cilantro
Shopping List	Fresh corn or canned corn, littleneck clams,carrots,celery,onion,thyme,chicken broth,heavy cream,salt, butter,1 hot pepper, olive oil, cilantro
Suggestions and Substitutions	This is very filling dish. Use it as a main meal. Use coconut cream for non-dairy substitute
Preparation	1. If fresh corn on the cob is used, cut each ear crosswise into thirds. Set aside. 2. Rinse the clams well and put them in a kettle. 3. Cut the carrot lengthwise in half. Cut each half crosswise into thin slices. There should be about one cup. Add this to the clams.

4. Coarsely chop the celery. There should be about one cup. Add this to the clams.

5. Coarsely chop the onion. There should be about one and one-half cups. Add the onion, thyme and wine to the clams.

6. Put the kettle over high heat and cover with a lid. Bring to the boil and cook until clams open, about three minutes.

7. Line another kettle with a sieve and line the sieve with cheesecloth. Or use a sieve of the sort known in French kitchens as a chinois.

8. Pour the clams, vegetables and liquid into the sieve. There should be about two and one-half cups of liquid. Add chicken broth to the clam liquid and bring to boil.

9. Meanwhile, remove the meat from the clams and set aside. Unless the meat pieces are small, cut the pieces in half. Discard the shells.

10. Add the strained vegetables to the clam and chicken broth. If corn on the cob is used, add it to the kettle and cook for about five minutes and add four cups of the cream. Bring to the boil. Add salt and pepper and let simmer for about 20 minutes.

11. If corn on the cob has been used, remove the pieces of corn from the kettle, using a pair of tongs. When the pieces of corn are cool enough to handle, cut the kernels from the cobs. There should be about five cups. Add this or the canned or frozen corn to the kettle. Pour the mixture,

one portion at a time, into the container of a food processor or, preferably, an electric blender and blend. Combine the blended soup in a kettle and add one tablespoon of lime juice, salt and pepper. There should be about 16 cups of soup. Add the meat from the clams.

12. Bring the soup to boil and swirl in the butter.

13. Chop the peppers coarsely. There should be about three tablespoons. Put the peppers in the container of an electric blender. Add the remaining lime juice, olive oil, cilantro, salt and pepper. Blend as fine as possible. This is to be used as a garnish for the soup.

14. Whip the remaining one cup of cream and add the blended

	pepper and lime juice mixture. Blend well.
	15. Serve the hot soup in 12 individual bowls and top each serving with an equal portion of the whipped cream mixture.
Suggested Spice, Side or Condiment	Corn Bread

Meal # 45 (once per week)	"Vermont Chicken Dinner"
	Cheddar garlic Crusted Chicken Breast with Sweet Yammys and Steamed Broccoli
Ingredients	**INGREDIENTS** ○ 1/3 cup butter, melted ○ 2 tablespoons minced garlic (can use more or less) ○ 2 teaspoons of garlic powder, divided (garlic lovers can use more) ○ 1/2 teaspoon seasoning salt (or can use white salt) ○ 3/4 cup seasoned dry bread crumb (seasoned or plain) ○ 1/2 cup finely grated cheddar cheese ○ 1/4 cup freshly grated parmesan cheese

	<ul><li>1/2 teaspoon ground black pepper (or to taste)</li><li>4 boneless skinless chicken breasts</li><li>shredded cheddar cheese (optional and use any amount desired, or can use shredded mozzarella cheese)</li></ul>
Shopping List	Butter, Garlic, Bread Crumbs, Free Range Chicken Breast, Shredded Cheddar Cheese, Parmesan, Sweet Potatoes

Meal # 46 (2 tacos)	"World's Best Fish Tacos" Fried Cod, Corn Avocado Salsa, Chipotle Vegan Mayo
Ingredients	6 oz fresh cod
	4 oz corn avocado salsa
	4 oz spring mix greens
	½ cup peanut oil
	2 6-inch whole wheat tortilla
	1 oz chipotle mayo
	¼ Red Onion
	¼ Jalapeno
	½ Juice Of Lime
	½ cup Chopped Cilantro
	Salt
	½ Tablespoon Vinegar
Substitutions	Flounder, Tuna, Grouper, Striped Bass, rainbow Trout, Catfish
Shopping List	6 oz fresh cod, Avocado, Fresh Corn, Bag spring mix greens,

	peanut oil, 6-inch whole wheat tortilla, vegan mayo, chipotle seasoning, fresh jalapeno, lime, cilantro, white vinegar,red onion, fish fry
Preparation	Slice cod into finger sized pieces Cut 1 avocado into 1 inch squares, dice ¼ red onion, diced 1 fresh jalapeno very small, Slice kernels off the corn, and combine it with all remaining ingredients in a bowl. Cover and refrigerate before serving. Slice kernels off the corn, and combine it with all remaining ingredients in a bowl. Cover and refrigerate before serving. In a medium deep frying pan add ½ cup peanut oil to hot pan

	Dredge cod in fish fry mixture and fry until golden brown. Drain on paper towels.
	Layer into 2 tortillas; Spring mix, Avocado Salsa, 3 pieces of fried cod, chipotle mayo
Suggested Spice, Side or Condiment	Chipotle Vegan Mayo

Meal # 47 (only once per week)	"The Mob Hit" Steak and Brooklyn Mashed Potatoes and Spinach
Ingredients	6-8oz Filet Mignon, 4 oz Spinach, 1 Potato, Butter, Salt and Pepper
Substitutions	*Ribeye or any lean beef preferable grain fed and organic*
Shopping List	6-8oz Filet mignon, baby spinach, idaho potatoes, butter
Suggestions	Save this as a restaurant meal if you are going out. Remember to plan ahead and check menu
Preparation	Prepare mashed potato as per side "Brooklyn Mashed"
Cooking Instructions	Grill or broil filet to desired temperature

	Saute spinach in peanut oil and garlic, drain oil
Suggested Spice, Side or Condiment	Vegan BBQ Sauce or Steak Sauce

Meal # 48 (4 portions)	"East End Mac and Cheese"
	Broccoli and Tomato mac and Cheese
Ingredients	½ head of broccoli, cut into small florets
	1 pint cherry tomatoes
	3 tablespoons olive oil
	Kosher salt and black pepper
	6 ounces whole wheat penne or shells
	¼ cup all-purpose flour
	2 cups low-fat milk
	4 ounces Cheddar

	2 ounces thinly sliced pepper jack cheese
Substitutions	*Grilled Vegetables*
Preparation	Cut broccoli into small florets Cut cherry tomatoes in half
Cooking Instructions	Heat oven to 425° F. Toss the broccoli, tomatoes,1 tablespoon of the oil, and 1/4 teaspoon each salt and pepper on a rimmed baking sheet. Roast, tossing once, until tender, 14 to 16 minutes. Remove from oven. Meanwhile, cook the pasta according to the package directions; drain. Heat the remaining 2 tablespoons of oil in a medium pot over medium heat. Add the flour and cook, whisking, for 30 seconds, Slowly

whisk in the milk. Cook, stirring occasionally, until thickened, 5 to 7 minutes. Remove from heat and stir in the Cheddar, vegetables, and pasta.

Transfer the mixture to a 2-quart baking dish. Top with pepper jack and broil until golden brown, 2 to 3 minutes.

Meal # 49	"Farmer's Margarita Pizza" Cauliflower Crust Pizza
Ingredients	1 small head cauliflower, stalk removed ½ cup shredded mozzarella 1/4 cup grated Parmesan 1/2 teaspoon dried oregano 1/2 teaspoon kosher salt 1/4 teaspoon garlic powder 2 eggs, lightly beaten
Time	1 hour
Preparation	Chop cauliflower into small florets and mix in a food processor until fine, Steam or boil until fully cooked and drain well.
Cooking Instructions	Preheat the oven to 400 degrees F. Line a baking sheet with parchment paper.

	In a bowl, combine the cauliflower with mozzarella, Parmesan, oregano, salt, garlic powder and eggs. Transfer to the center of the baking sheet and spread into a circle, resembling a pizza crust. Bake for 20 minutes. Add fresh mozzarella, plum tomatoes and basil leaves and bake an additional 10 minutes.
Suggested Spice, Side or Condiment	Fresh parmesan

Meal # 50	"Twisted Sin" Veggie Pasta with garlic and oil
Ingredients	1 Yellow Squash 1 Green Squash 1 Clove garlic 1 oz fresh parsley Salt and pepper to taste 1 oz olive oil
Substitutions	*Any vegetable that can be sliced thin in a string similar to pasta. Any squash, Eggplant.*
Suggestions	Use "Veggetti" or other type of vegetable slicer that can slice vegetables into long strings
Preparation	Cut ends off of squash, Slice into pasta shape. Smash and chop garlic
Cooking Instructions	Heat saute pan Add olive oil and garlic

	As soon as garlic begins to cook add vegetable pasta. Toss and saute for 5 minutes or until vegetable pasta is tender. Tip: add a ¼ cup water to slow cooking
Suggested Spice, Side or Condiment	Fresh pecorino romano cheese and a piece of whole grain bread.

Meal # 51	Mario's Linguine and Clam Sauce
Ingredients	12 Top neck clams 1 clove garlic 2 oz fresh parsley 2 oz olive oil ½ pint clam juice Gluten Free or Whole Wheat Linguine
Suggestions	Where a bib
Preparation	Shuck 1 dozen top neck clams. Scoop out meat and save broth. Smash and Chop 1 clove garlic Wash and chop parsley Mix all ingredients with clam juice and olive oil and let sit for 4-6 hours.
Cooking Instructions	Cook pasta al dente Put sauce in saute pan and heat until broth starts to bubble. Add ¼ lb cooked pasta to pan, toss and serve

Suggested Spice, Side or Condiment	Top with pecorino romano cheese and serve with whole grain bread so soak up broth.

Meal # 52	Hot Summer Nights Lobster Salad Sandwich
Ingredients	¼ Lb. Lobster tail and claw meat ½ cup vegan mayo ½ Cup celery Pinch salt and pepper to taste Juice of 1 lemon Whole Grain Bread or Roll
Substitutions	*Shrimp, Crawfish*
Suggestions	Have over bed of lettuce instead of bread
Preparation	Chop lobster into small chunks Dice celery Squeeze juice out of lemon
Instructions	Mix lemon and lobster meat first then add mayonnaise, salt and pepper and mix well.
Suggested Spice, Side or Condiment	Cholula Hot Sauce

Sides and Condiments

Side # 1	**"Pablo Escobar's Favorite Salsa"**
Ingredients	2-3 medium sized fresh tomatoes (from 1 lb to 1 1/2 lb), stems removed. 1. 1/2 red onion. 2. 2 serrano chiles or 1 jalapeño chile (stems, ribs, seeds removed), less or more to taste. 3. Juice of one lime. 4. 1/2 cup chopped cilantro. 5. Salt and pepper to taste.
Substitutions	*Peppers, mango,*
Suggestions	Do not contact the family for recipe tips!
Preparation	Dice tomatoes, onions and chiles. Mix all ingredients. Let stand for 1 hour.

Side # 2	"Backyard BBQ Sauce"
Ingredients	1/4 cup molasses 1/8 cup apple cider vinegar 2 tablespoons olive oil 1/2 cup dark purple jam such as blueberry or blackberry 1/4 cup maple syrup or agave 1 tablespoon shoyu sauce (or soy sauce) 2 cloves garlic – minced or pressed 1 tablespoon smoked paprika 1 tablespoon dried oregano (use more if fresh) two dashes hot sauce (or more to taste) fresh cracked pepper to taste

Preparation	Whisk together until fully combined. Put in a saucepan, cover and simmer for 20 minutes on LOW.

Side # 3	"Happy Ketchup"
Ingredients	• 1 (6 ounce) Can of Tomato Paste • ¾ – 1 Cup Water (thin to desired consistency) • 2 Tablespoons Sugar (Evaporated Cane Juice, Date Sugar, etc...) • 2 Tablespoons Apple Cider Vinegar • ½ Teaspoon Salt • ¼ Teaspoon Onion Powder • ¼ Teaspoon Garlic Powder • ¼ Teaspoon Mustard Powder • Pinch of Ground Cinnamon • Pinch of Ground Cloves • Pinch of Ground Allspice

	• Pinch of Cayenne Pepper (or to taste)
Preparation	Whisk all ingredients together in saucepan until mixed well and smooth. For an even smoother consistency, you can blend all of the ingredients in your Vitamix before heating.

Add extra water 1 Tablespoon at a time if necessary until you have the desired consistency. We like our Ketchup a little thinner, and it thickens a small amount as it cools.

Cook on Medium Heat until Ketchup is hot and bubbles begin to break at the surface. Stir constantly for 1-2 minutes and remove from heat.

Allow Ketchup to cool completely before placing in airtight container |

	Store in airtight container for 1-2 months in Fridge.

Side # **4**	**"Girly Mayo"**
Ingredients	8 ounces silken tofu
	2 to 3 tablespoons neutral-tasting vegetable oil, like grapeseed or canola
	1 to 2 tablespoons lemon juice or cider vinegar
	1/2 teaspoon salt
	1 teaspoon dijon or yellow mustard, optional
	1/2 teaspoon agave nectar or other sweetener, if you like a slightly sweet mayonnaise
Preparation	1. Drain and rinse the tofu: Very gently drain the tofu and rinse under running water. It's fine if it breaks while

you're rinsing. Transfer the tofu to a blender, a food processor, or the cup of an immersion blender.

2. Combine the mayo ingredients: Add the oil, vinegar, and salt to the tofu. Start with the lesser of the recommended amounts; you can add more to taste later on.

3. Blend until smooth and creamy: Blend the tofu continuously until it becomes smooth and very creamy. Stop the blender and scrape down the sides as needed during blending.

4. Taste and adjust: Taste the mayonnaise. Add more olive oil for a creamier, richer mayo or a tablespoon of water to loosen the texture. Add mustard or agave, additional

	lemon juice or vinegar, or more salt, according to your taste.
	5. Use or store the mayo: Store the mayonnaise in the refrigerator for up to one week.

Side # 5 (4-6 servings)	"Hummus of the Gods"
Ingredients	1 15-ounce can chickpeas or 1 1/2 cups cooked chickpeas 1/4 cup fresh lemon juice 1/4 cup well-stirred tahini 1 small garlic clove, minced 2 tablespoons extra-virgin olive oil, plus more for serving 1/2 teaspoon ground cumin Salt to taste 2 to 3 tablespoons water Dash ground paprika, for serving
Suggestions	*If you are cheese lover keep a lot of hummus around. It's a good substitute.*
Preparation	**Prepare the Hummus:** In the bowl of a food processor, combine the

tahini and lemon juice and process for 1 minute, scraping the sides and bottom of the bowl then process for 30 seconds more.

This extra time helps "whip" or "cream" the tahini, making the hummus smooth and creamy.

Add the olive oil, minced garlic, cumin, and a 1/2 teaspoon of salt to the whipped tahini and lemon juice. Process for 30 seconds, scrape the sides and bottom of the bowl then process another 30 seconds or until well blended.

Add chickpeas: Open, drain and rinse the chickpeas. Add half of the chickpeas to the food processor and process for 1 minute. Scrape sides and bottom of the bowl, then add remaining chickpeas and process until thick and quite smooth; 1 to 2 minutes.

	Create the Perfect Consistency: Most likely the hummus will be too thick or still have tiny bits of chickpea. To fix this, with the food processor turned on, slowly add 2 to 3 tablespoons of water until you reach the perfect consistency.

Meal # 6	What in the World is Tahini?
Ingredients	<ul><li>1 cup (5 ounces or 140 grams) sesame seeds, we prefer hulled</li><li>3 to 4 tablespoons neutral flavored oil such as grapeseed, canola or a light olive oil</li><li>Pinch of salt, optional</li></ul>
Preparation	**Toast Sesame Seeds (optional):** Add sesame seeds to a wide, dry saucepan over medium-low heat and toast, stirring constantly until the seeds become fragrant and very lightly colored (not brown), 3 to 5 minutes. Transfer toasted seeds to a baking sheet or large plate and

cool completely. (Careful here, sesame seeds can burn quickly).

Make Tahini Paste: Add sesame seeds to the bowl of a food processor then process until a crumbly paste forms, about 1 minute. Add 3 tablespoons of the oil then process for 2 to 3 minutes more, stopping to scrape the bottom and sides of the food processor a couple times. Check the tahini consistency. It should be smooth, not gritty and should be pourable. You may need to process for another minute or add the additional tablespoon of oil.

Taste the tahini for seasoning then add salt to taste. Process 5 to 10 seconds to mix it in.

Side # 7 (4-6 servings)	1-2-3 **Guacamole**
Ingredients	2 avocados 2 tablespoons minced onion 2 tablespoons lime juice, or more to taste ¼ teaspoon sea salt, or more to taste ½ cup cilantro 1 cup chopped tomato
Substitutions	*Great snack food*
Preparation	Combine the onion, lime juice and salt in a medium bowl. Peel and pit the avocados and add to the bowl.

	Mash with potato masher until combined. Taste and add more lime juice and salt if needed.
Suggested Spice, Side or Condiment	Black Bean Chips

Side # 8 (8-10 servings)	"Mashed Sweet Yammy's"
Ingredients	6 sweet potatoes, peeled and cubed 3/4 cup almond milk 1/2 cup butter 3/4 cup real maple syrup
Suggestions	Great to keep around for up to a week. Use as a side for dinner meals or as a snack.
Preparation	Bring a large pot of salted water to boil. Add potatoes and cook until tender, 20 to 30 minutes. With an electric mixer on low, blend potatoes, slowly adding milk, about 1/2 a cup at a time. Use more or less to achieve desired texture. Add butter and maple syrup to taste. Blend until smooth. Serve warm.
Suggested Spice, Side or Condiment	Cholula, Almond Butter

Side # 9 (6-8 servings)	"Brooklyn Mashed Potatoes"
Ingredients	<ul><li>2 lb. Idaho potatoes</li><li>3 tbsp. Kosher salt</li><li>1 c. almond milk</li><li>4 tbsp. cold almond butter</li><li>½ tsp. fresh-ground black pepper</li></ul>
Preparation	Peel potatoes and cut into small cubes
Cooking Instructions	Boil potatoes until fork tender. Drain and return to pot. Add all other ingredients and mash with a potato masher.
Suggested Spice, Side or Condiment	Vegan Ketchup

Side # 10	"The Sauce"
Ingredients	1 tablespoon olive oil
	1/2 red onion, small dice
	4 tablespoons minced garlic
	Salt and freshly ground black pepper
	6 fresh basil leaves, chopped
	3 tablespoons red wine
	1 (28-ounce) can whole plum tomatoes

	1/2 cup water
Preparation	Heat the oil in a pot over medium heat. Add the onion and garlic and cook for about 5 to 7 minutes, until onions are soft and translucent. Season with salt and pepper, to taste, and add the basil leaves, red wine, and tomatoes. Bring to a boil, then simmer for about 20 to 25 minutes.

Barret's Diet Plan Shopping Checklist

Take an inventory at home and fill out column 1 before you go shopping. This will also help you mentally prepare your meals while you are shopping.

Item	Stocked at home	Need to buy
Sample item		
Free Range Eggs	¼ box	1 box
Egg Whites	½ quart	1 quart

Breads

We have been fooled into believing that we have limited options for bread if we trust what the supermarket sells us. Why do we have a bread "aisle" and a bakery "section". Should be called the "convenience" aisle and the "better stuff" section. There are so many beautiful, delicious, healthy whole grain, whole wheat, and rye bread available on the market. The key is to watch out for unbleached flour, sodium content, and saturated fat. Package must say 100% whole grain or 100% whole wheat or 100% rye. For the Barretts diet plan we recommend sticking to whole grain because it's loaded with nutrients and fiber. Do your research. If you have a good local bakery the baker would be happy to tell you the ingredients as well. Ask around. People love good bread.

Here are the 7 healthiest breads you can choose according to Healthline.com

1. Sprouted **whole grain**. Sprouted bread is made from whole grains that have started to sprout from exposure to heat and moisture. ...
2. Sourdough. ...
3. 100% whole wheat. ...
4. Oat bread. ...
5. Flax bread. ...
6. 100% sprouted rye bread. ...
7. Healthy gluten-free bread.

https://www.healthline.com/nutrition/healthiest-bread#section1

Tips for Choosing Vegetables at the Market

• **Cabbages:** Choose firm, compact heads that feel heavy for their size. Check that the stems are also fresh and compact.

• **Carrots:** Choose firm, smooth carrots without rootlets.

• **Cauliflower:** Choose heads with tightly packed, creamy white florets. Avoid yellowed, spotted, or flowering florets.

• **Celery:** Choose firm, unblemished stalks. The stalks and leaves should be green, not yellow.

• **Celery Root:** Choose firm, hard roots that feel heavy for their size. Any attached leaves should be fresh and green.

• **Corn:** Choose corn with bright green husks and moist but not slimy silk. Peel back the husk to ensure the kernels are plump and not dry.

• **Cucumbers:** Choose cucumbers that are uniformly green (not yellow).

• **Eggplants:** Choose eggplants that have smooth, naturally shiny skin and feel heavy for their size. When gently pressed, flesh that gives slightly and then bounces back indicates ripeness.

- **Artichokes:** Choose globes that have tight leaves and feel heavy for their size. The leaves should squeak when pressed against each other.

- **Asparagus:** Choose firm, smooth, and brightly-colored stalks with compact tips. Avoid limp stalks. Choose stalks of equal thickness to ensure even cooking times.

- **Avocados:** Choose avocados that feel slightly soft to the touch. Firmer avocados may be ripened at home, but avoid rock-hard ones. Also avoid avocados with cracks or dents.

- **Beets:** Choose firm beets with fresh stems and slender taproots. Avoid beets with wilted leaves, scaly tops, or large, hairy taproots as they may be older and more woody.

- **Bok Choy:** For mature bok choy, look for dark green leaves and bright white stalks. Baby bok choy should be light green in color.

- **Broccoli:** Choose broccoli with firm stalks, tight florets, and crisp green leaves. Avoid yellowed or flowering florets.

- **Brussels Sprouts:** Choose firm, compact, bright green heads. Avoid sprouts with wilted or loose outer leaves.

Eggplants: Skin will not give, while overripe flesh will remain indented. Also, smaller eggplants tend to have fewer seeds and be less bitter.

• **Fennel:** Choose fennel with white, firm, unblemished bulbs as well as firm stems and fresh leaves.

• **Garlic:** Choose firm, plump heads. Avoid heads with soft spots or green sprouts.

• **Green Beans:** Choose slender beans that snap rather than bend. Avoid bulging or dried pods.

• **Jerusalem Artichokes:** Choose smooth, firm tubers. Avoid those with green spots or sprouts.

• **Kale:** Choose crisp, deeply-colored leaves. Avoid yellowed leaves. Smaller leaves tend to be more tender.

• **Leeks:** Choose firm leeks with tightly-rolled tops. Slender leeks tend to be younger and more tender, while larger ones with rounded bulbs tend to be older and more woody.

- **Lettuce, Spinach, and Other Leafy Greens:** Choose greens with fresh, crisp leaves. Avoid any that are wilted or slimy.

- **Onions and Shallots:** Choose dry, firm bulbs that feel heavy for their size. Avoid any with soft spots or green sprouts.

- **Parsnips:** Choose firm, ivory-colored roots. Large roots may be fibrous, so choose small and medium ones for better texture and flavor.

- **Peas:** Choose crisp, green pods. Avoid bulging, dried, yellow, or white pods.

- **Peppers:** Choose firm, naturally shiny peppers that feel heavy for their size.

- **Potatoes:** Choose firm, smooth potatoes. Avoid those with bruises, green spots, or sprouts.

- **Radishes:** Choose radishes with fresh, green tops and firm, unblemished roots.

- **Rhubarb:** Choose firm pink or red stalks. Green stalks tend to be stringy and sour.

- **Rutabagas:** Choose rutabagas that feel firm and heavy for their size. Avoid any with holes or bruises.

- **Scallions:** Choose scallions with crisp, green tops and firm, white bulbs. Avoid wilted or browned scallions.

- **Summer Squash:** Choose squash with naturally shiny, taught, unblemished skin. Avoid squash that appear dull or have soft spots.

- **Sweet Potatoes and Yams:** Choose potatoes with firm, unwrinkled skin and no bruises or cuts, as they are highly perishable.

- **Swiss Chard:** Choose chard with crisp stalks and shiny, bright, unwilted leaves.

- **Tomatillos:** Choose green tomatillos with green husks. Avoid yellow fruits with brown husks.

- **Tomatoes:** Choose tomatoes that are fragrant, smell earthy at the stem end, and feel heavy for their size. Avoid tomatoes with wrinkled skin.

- **Turnips:** Choose turnips that feel firm and heavy for their size. Smaller turnips **tend to be sweeter and more tender than larger ones, which may be woody.**

- **Winter Squash:** Choose squash that have stems intact and feel heavy for their size. Avoid squash with cuts or soft spots.

Fish Buying Tips

Fresh Fish

Fresh, unfrozen fish smells like seawater or cucumber. If it gives off a strong, objectionable odor, it's past its prime. Finfish should have firm, elastic flesh that is unmarred. Any exposed flesh should appear freshly cut without traces of browning or drying out. The skin should be moist with unfaded characteristic markings and the colors of that species. If the fish has scales, they should adhere closely to the skin and should not be dry or look "ruffled". If you press on the fish the flesh should bounce back and not leave an indentation. Plan to use fresh fish within two days of purchase. Maximum quality in fresh fish is maintained if fish is loosely wrapped and packed in finely crushed ice to prevent moisture loss. If you are unable to use the fish within two days, go ahead and cook or freeze it. Cooked fish maintains quality in the refrigerator at 32-34°F for two to three days. (See information below about freezing fish.)

Clams and Mussels

These mollusks should be alive when sold. It's easy to tell if they are alive because their shells will be closed. If the shells are gaping open, give them a quick tap: this will prompt live clams and mussels to tightly close their shells. They will also give off a sweet smell. Mollusks should be iced or refrigerated between 34-40°F. At home, store them dry and uncovered in a pot or bowl in the refrigerator. Be sure they have room to breathe — never store them in a plastic bag where they will suffocate. Ideally, purchase mollusks from a fish market that stores them in saltwater tanks.

Oysters

Fresh oysters are sold shucked or in the shell. Oysters must be alive if purchased in the shell, indicated by shells that close tightly when handled. Live oysters are sold by the dozen or by the bag containing approximately one bushel. Live oysters will remain alive for 7 to 10 days if stored without ice in the refrigerator at 35-40°F. Shucked oysters are graded and sold according to size, usually in pints or gallons. Fresh shucked oysters are plump and have a natural creamy color and clear liquid. If properly handled and packed in ice in the refrigerator, freshly shucked oysters will maintain quality for about a week. We don't recommend that you freeze oysters at home, simply because they freeze too slowly in a home freezer to produce a satisfactory product.

Shrimp

Only two percent of shrimp is sold fresh, and most is sold within 50 miles of the coast. Fresh shrimp maintain a firm texture and mild odor. Remember that raw, headless shrimp in the shell maintain quality during freezing longer than frozen, cooked shrimp and are best if frozen at the peak of freshness.

Lobsters

Live lobsters should be active and should curl their tails under when picked up. They should be aggressive in their movements.

Crab

Fresh hard-shelled crabs are sold either alive, or as cooked meat (fresh or pasteurized). If you purchase live crabs, make sure they show movement. Fresh soft-shell crabs should have a moist appearance and be free of odor. Fresh or pasteurized crabmeat has a very mild odor and should be used within one to two days of purchase. It will maintain quality better if packed in ice in the refrigerator. Pasteurized crab meat must be kept

under refrigeration, just like fresh crab meat.

Fish

Low-fat Fish

Fish are one of the best sources of the essential omega-3 fats eicosapentaenoic acid, or EPA, and docosahexaenoic acid, or DHA. These omega-3 fats may lower your risk for heart disease, which is why the American Heart Association recommends you eat fish at least twice a week. Low-fat fish make it easier to stay within the recommended fat limit for the day of no more than 35 percent of your calories, but may also be lower in essential omega-3 fats than higher-fat fish.

The fish that provide the least amount of fat, with less than 2 grams of fat per 3-ounces of cooked fish, including orange roughy, tuna, pollock, mahi mahi, cod, hake, haddock, sole and flounder. Tuna and cod are especially good options if you are trying to maximize your protein intake, since they are among the fish highest in protein per calorie. Choose tuna or pollock if you are trying to maximize your omega-3 fats while minimizing total fat consumption.

Tilapia, chum and pink salmon, ocean perch, halibut and Pacific rockfish are also low in fat, with less than 5 grams of fat per 3 ounces of cooked fish. Of these options, salmon is significantly higher in omega-3 fats, providing 900 to 1,825 milligrams per serving depending on the type you choose. This is more than the recommended amount of at least 500 milligrams per day.

Additional Low-fat Seafood Options

While not technically fish, shrimp, scallops, crabs, lobsters and clams all contain less than 2 grams of fat per 3-ounce serving and oysters and mussels provide less than 5 grams per serving. Oysters, crab and scallops all provide at least 300 milligrams of omega-3 fats per serving, making them among the best low-fat seafood choices.

Other Fish Health Considerations

When choosing fish or seafood, fat content isn't the only important factor. Some types of seafood tend to contain higher levels of mercury than others, making it important to limit these in your diet. Orange roughy, big eye and ahi tuna are among the low-fat fish highest in mercury, so avoid these. Yellowfin and canned albacore tuna are also high in mercury, so choose chunk light tuna or skipjack tuna instead. The fish both lowest in fat and lowest in mercury include flounder, hake and haddock. Salmon, tilapia, ocean perch, shrimp, scallops, crabs and clams are also good low-fat and low-mercury options.

Organic food Purchasing Guidelines

What do the food labels such as "organic," "natural," "free-range," and "non-GMO" really mean? Understanding this terminology is essential when you're shopping for organic food.

The most important point to remember is that "natural" does not equal organic. "Natural" or "all natural" on packaged food are unregulated terms that can be applied by anyone, whereas organic certification means that set production standards have been met. These production standards vary from country to country—in the U.S., for example, only the "USDA Organic" label indicates that a food is certified organic. Similar certification labels are also offered on organic products in other parts of the world, including the European Union, Canada, and Australia.

USDA certified organic food labels in the U.S.

When you're shopping for organic foods in the U.S., look for the "USDA Organic" seal. Only foods that are 95 to 100 percent organic (and GMO-free) can use the USDA Organic label.

- **100% Organic** – Foods that are completely organic or made with 100% organic ingredients may display the USDA seal.

- **Organic** – Foods that contain at least 95% organic ingredients may display the USDA seal.

- **Made with organic ingredients** – Foods that contain at least 70% organic ingredients will not display the USDA seal but may list specific organic ingredients on the front of the package.

- **Contains organic ingredients** – Foods that contain less than 70% organic ingredients will not display the USDA seal but may list specific organic ingredients on the information panel of the package.

Certified Organic and Small Farms

Keep in mind that even if a producer is certified organic in the U.S., the use of the USDA Organic label is voluntary. At the same time, not everyone goes through the rigorous process of becoming certified, especially smaller farming operations. When shopping at a farmers' market, for example, don't hesitate to ask the vendors how their food was grown.

Non-GMO labels

Genetically Modified Organisms (GMOs) or genetically engineered (GE) foods are plants or animals whose DNA has been altered in ways that cannot occur in nature or in traditional crossbreeding, most commonly in order to be resistant to pesticides or produce an insecticide. The introduction of GMOs has had a profound effect on the level of pesticides present on and in our food, and potentially on our health and the environment.

In the U.S., GMOs are commonly found in crops such as soybeans, alfalfa, squash, zucchini, papaya, and canola, and are present in many breakfast cereals and much of the processed food that we eat. If the ingredients on a package include corn syrup or soy lecithin, chances are it contains GMOs.

Shopping for non-GMO foods

In most countries, organic crops contain no GMOs and organic meat comes from animals raised on organic, GMO-free feed.

When shopping for GMO-free food products in the U.S. and Canada, look for the Non-GMO Project Verified seal, which means that no more than 0.9% of the product is genetically engineered. See the Resources section below for a database of foods verified as non-GMO, available online and in a smartphone app.

Foods labeled "GMO free" or "Non-GMO" *– Without the seal, foods labeled with these terms have NOT necessarily undergone independent verification.*

Meat and dairy labels

In the U.S., the organic label is the most regulated term, but when it comes to meat we often see many other terms used. In order to make informed choices, it is helpful to know what some of these terms mean.

- **Natural or all natural** – This label means "minimally processed" and that the meat can't have any artificial colors, artificial flavors, preservatives, or any other artificial ingredients in it. Animals can still be given antibiotics or growth enhancers and meat can be injected with salt, water, and other ingredients. For example, this term can be applied to all raw cuts of beef since they aren't processed. The natural label does **not** reflect how the animal was raised or fed, which makes it fairly meaningless.

- **Naturally raised** – This claim should be followed by a specific statement, such as "naturally raised without antibiotics or growth hormones" in order to obtain USDA approval. Read different labels carefully to understand what naturally raised really means to the piece of meat you're buying.

- **Grass-fed** – This term claims that the animals are fed solely on a diet of grass or hay and have continuous access to the outdoors. Cattle are naturally ruminants that eat grass, so they tend to be healthier and leaner when fed this way. In addition, grass fed beef has been shown to have more of the healthy omega-3 fatty acids. However, if meat is labeled as grass fed but **not** certified organic, the animal may have been raised on pasture that was exposed to or treated with synthetic pesticides or fertilizers.

- **Free-range** or free-roaming – Broadly, this term means that the animals weren't confined to a cage and had access to the outdoors. Unfortunately, there are no requirements for the amount of time the animals spend outdoors or for the size of the outdoor space available. The terms free-range or free-roaming also don't apply to egg-laying hens. While it's difficult to tell exactly what free range means on meat packaging, you can contact the producer directly for clarification.

- **Cage-free** – The term means that egg-laying hens are not raised in cages. However, it does not necessarily mean they have access to the outdoors. Some eggs may carry the American Humane Certified label but many cage-free claims are not certified, making it a very misleading label.

- **Pasture-raised** – This claims that the animals were not raised in confinement and had year-round access to the outside. Again, there are no requirements for exactly how much time the animals spend outside or the size of the outdoor space available, so it can be misleading.

- **No hormones added or hormone-free** – This term indicates that animals are raised without the use of any added growth hormones. For beef and dairy products, it can be helpful, but by law in the U.S., poultry, veal calves, and pigs cannot be given hormones, so don't pay extra for chicken, veal, or pork products that use this label.

- **Certified Humane Raised and Handled** – This is a voluntary certification regulated by the Humane Farm Animal Care, a non-profit organization aimed at ensuring the humane treatment of farm animals. The label means that animals have ample space, shelter, and gentle handling to limit stress, ample fresh water, and a diet without added antibiotics or hormones. Animals must be able to roam around and root without ever being confined to cages, crates, or tie stalls.

Glossary of Food Label and Organic Terms

Adulteration - The addition of a substance to an essential oil after distillation. This is generally done to make the final product greater in volume; being mixed with extraneous material.

Aloe Barbadensis (Aloe) Leaf Extract - Derived from the leaf; aloe is rich in vitamins, minerals, amino acids, enzymes, proteins, humectants, anti-inflammatory and antibacterial properties. Aloe nourishes and protects the skin.

Alternative Therapy - Complementary medicinal disciplines that typically use natural, rather than chemical, approaches.

Aromatherapy - The art and science of using pure essential oils extracted from natural botanicals to relax, balance and rejuvenate the body, mind and spirit.

Aromatherapy Benefit - The emotional or physical effect evoked by aromatic essential oils. Examples include balancing, energizing, rejuvenating, cleansing, deodorizing and purifying.

Aromatic plant - A plant that produces essential oils and has a distinct and unique smell.

Artificial flavor - The United States Code of Federal Regulations (21 CFR 102.22) defines "artificial flavors" as any substance with the purpose of imparting flavor that is not derived from an herb, spice, fruit, vegetable, or other plant or animal source.

Attar - A term, first used in the 18th Century, for perfume or essential oil obtained from flowers or petals, as in "attar of roses" for rose oil.

Autolyzed yeast - Yeast extracts are carefully fermented from cane and/or beet molasses and are autolyzed by enzymes under exacting conditions. Autolysis is the destruction of tissues or cells of an organism by substances, such as enzymes. By varying the fermentation and autolysis conditions, several unique flavor enhancers can be made. Don't confuse this product with active yeast or nutritional yeast.

Avena Sativa (Oat) Kernel Powder - Ground from the whole grain containing all of the natural counter-irritants and skin soothing properties that oat is known for.

Ayurveda - A system of traditional medicine established in India over 3,000 years ago — literally the "science of life." Ayurveda includes food, exercise, meditation, detoxification, hygiene, massage and ethical conduct, as well as natural vegetable medicines in its practice. Herbs are used as special foods to help bring the individual back to a state of harmony by eliminating excesses and strengthening in areas of deficiencies. Ayurveda recognizes three body types or doshas — vata (air) is dry, light, cold, hard and clear, pitta (fire and water) is hot, fluid, light, subtle and sharp, and kapha (earth and water) is cold, wet, slow, heavy and dense. Treatments include understanding the combination of the doshas in each person as well as the condition.

Base Notes - The aromatic components of essential oils that do not readily evaporate and are used as fixatives to provide permanence and stability.

Base oil - A vegetable oil. Also called a carrier oil or fixed oil.

Bay Laurel - Bay is sometimes called bay laurel or sweet bay in order to identify it as the spice from the *Laurus nobilis* tree. West Indian Bay, *Pimenta racemosa*, is the source of bay oil, an ingredient in bay rum. California bay, *Umbellularia californica*, is sometimes sold as bay leaf spice because of its very attractive appearance but it is not GRAS (generally recognized as safe for consumption by the FDA).

Bergapten - Many plants contain furocoumarins such as bergapten, which are known photosensitizers. Bergapten is a naturally occurring component of bergamot essential oil. When bergamot oil is applied, the skin can become very sensitive to ultraviolet light. Severity of the reaction depends on length of exposure and individual sensitivity. Mild cases can be a reddening of the skin, while severe cases can result in acute lesions known as bullock dermatitis. The dermatitis will resolve itself in a few weeks; however the accompanying hyperpigmentation (brown spots on the skin) can take months or years to fully disappear. Aura Cacia offers a bergaptene-free version of bergamot essential oil. There is no evidence to indicate that removing the bergapten in anyway affects the aromatherapy benefit of the essential oil and we recommend using bergaptene-free bergamot whenever possible.

Bioflavonoids - Bioflavonoids are any of a group of biologically active flavone compounds that may help maintain the capillary walls, reducing the likelihood of hemorrhaging. They are widely found in plants, especially citrus fruits. They are commonly added to Vitamin C for optimum absorption. They are used in our Vitamin C blend.

Bitters - The term bitters often refers to a bitter-tasting, unsweetened alcoholic beverage flavored with herbs and spices. Herbal bitters do not contain alcohol but are usually used similarly to the alcoholic versions — as a before- or after-dinner beverage. The sensation of bitter flavor in the mouth sends a message to the central nervous system that causes the body to begin to prepare itself for eating. Foods with a bitter flavor can also do the same thing — if you simply imagine biting into a lemon, you may find yourself starting to salivate. Formulas made from bitter herbs and spices have tonifying effects on the body and some people like to consume them daily. Herbs often used in herbal bitters include gentian, blessed thistle, goldenseal, bitter orange peel, wormwood, horehound, yarrow, dandelion, boneset, hops and artichoke leaf. Since the bitter flavor is what sends a signal to the brain, bitters must be tasted to be effective. While they should not be sweetened, spices such as cinnamon, cloves and allspice can be added to increase their warming effect and improve the flavor.

Black Tea - The most widely consumed teas, black teas are full-flavored and characterized by a tannic, woody astringency with subtle, flowery nuances. To make black tea, the leaves are picked and withered for one to two days and then rolled (rolling helps to release the enzymes needed for the next step). Next the leaves are oxidized, which develops the characteristic black tea flavor and changes the color of the leaves from green to brown or black. Finally, the tea is fired in ovens to stop oxidation and dry leaves.

Body (tea) - Body refers to the weight of prepared tea on the tongue. A tea can have a heavy, medium, full or light body.

Bone char - Bone char: Bone char, also known as animal charcoal or abaiser, is a granular material with high adsorption capacity produced by charring animal bones at high temperatures in an oxygen-depleted atmosphere. Bone char is used in applications such as defluoridation of water and removal of heavy metals from aqueous solutions. It's sometimes used in the sugar-refining industry for decolorizing. Bone char is not used in the production of our sugar or in the production of any sugar used as an ingredient in our products.

Boswellia Spp Resinoid - Derived from the resin of the frankincense tree. Balsamic, incense-like aroma. Centering and meditative.

Botanical Name - Refers to the Latin name of the plant in the biological classification system. A botanical name is composed of the genus followed by the species. It is the internationally recognized Latin name of a plant.

Bourbon Vanilla - Bourbon vanilla refers to vanilla grown on what used to be called the "Bourbon islands" - Madagascar, The Comoros, Reunion and the Seychelles. Located off the eastern coast of Africa, the Bourbon Islands were named for the French monarchy that ruled them at that time.

Broken Orange Pekoe (BOP) - Tea is graded by leaf size. Broken orange pekoe consists of broken and smaller sized leaves.

Bubble Tea - Bubble tea is a novel beverage gaining popularity in some parts of the country. It is made by pouring hot tea over cooked and cooled tapioca pearls. Any hot tea can be used. Bubble tea is served in a tall glass, usually with milk.

Butyrospermum Parkii (Shea) Nut Butter - Yellowish butter expelled from the nut-like fruit of the Karite tree of the Ivory Coast of Africa; shea butter adds a rich buttery consistency to the product while also providing relief for superficial irritation, dryness, dermatitis, eczema and other skin conditions.

CFR (Code of Federal Regulations) - The Code of Federal Regulations is an extensive compilation of all of the federal regulations. It is printed once a year and is also available electronically. The code is divided into titles, so for example title 21 covers all the food regulations. References to the code are made by first stating the title, then the name CFR, then the section and subsection.

CO2 Extraction - A method of extracting essential oil using liquid CO_2 as a solvent.

Calcium - Calcium is a mineral essential to human health. It is the most abundant mineral in the body, making up to 2% of total body weight with over 99% found in the bones. It is important in building and maintaining bones and teeth as well as playing a role in other functions such as muscle contraction, blood clotting and regulation of heartbeat. Foods abundant in calcium are dairy products, seaweed, dark leafy greens, tofu and nuts. If taking calcium supplements, chelated forms such as calcium citrate, calcium lactate or calcium gluconate are absorbed by the body more efficiently.

Calcium Silicate - Lime and diatomaceous earth. Absorbent. Bulking agent.

California Bay - California bay, *Umbellularia californica*, is a large, native tree often grown as an ornamental. The leaves are sometimes used in cooking as a replacement for bay laurel. Some spice companies like to sell it instead of true bay because the leaves are more attractive in a clear spice bottle. Unlike bay laurel, California bay is not GRAS (generally recognized as safe for consumption by the FDA) and if sold as bay leaf rather than under a different name, it is not in compliance with FDA regulations which have established a standard of identity for bay of *Laurus nobilis*. In addition, California bay contains umbellulone, a central nervous system toxin.

Camphoraceous - Being or having the properties of camphor.

Caprylic/Capric Triglyceride - A blend of three glycerides derived from coconut oil; assists in the solubilization of ingredients while acting as an emollient and skin lubricant.

Carbomer - Toxic-free synthetic ingredient; assists with thickening the product.

Carbon Dioxide Decaffeination - Carbon Dioxide (CO_2) Decaffeination - In the CO_2 decaffeination process, water soaked tea leaves are placed in a stainless steel container or extractor. The extractor is then sealed and liquid CO_2 is injected. The CO_2 acts as a solvent to dissolve and draw the caffeine from the leaves, leaving the larger-molecule flavor components behind. The caffeine laden CO_2 is then transferred to another container. Here the pressure is released and the CO_2 returns to its gaseous state, leaving the caffeine behind. The caffeine free CO_2 gas is pumped back into a pressurized container for reuse. CO_2 decaffeination produces the most flavorful decaffeinated tea. There are no harmful chemicals or byproducts of the process.

Cardamom Pods, White - White cardamom pods are bleached with sulfur to turn the green pods white. White cardamoms are preferred in some countries, especially in Europe, although the flavor and aroma of the seeds is adversely affected. Frontier does not sell white cardamon because of the residual sulfur levels on the product.

Carrageenan - Carrageenan is a water-soluble substance extracted from red seaweed, mainly *Chondrus crispus* or Irish Moss. Carrageenan is used in both cosmetic and food applications as a stabilizer and emulsifier capable of controlling viscosity, maintaining product integrity, and for giving an improved mouthfeel and body to foods. Carrageenan is a commonly used ingredient in dry mixes, desserts, milk products, tomato sauces, salad dressings and cheese products. To extract carrageenan at home, boil a quantity of Irish moss wrapped in cheesecloth for a short period of time. Carrageenan will be extracted from the seaweed and into the water. Upon cooling the liquid will form a soft gel.

Carrier - A substance used to dilute essential oils.

Certified Organic Farming - Cultivation without the use of artificial herbicides, fertilizers or pesticides. Certification by an independent third party ensures the plants are grown, harvested, transported and processed in ways that protect their integrity.

Cetyl Alcohol - Derived from coconut and/or palm kernel oil ; the dry, waxlike fatty alcohol acts as a co-emulsifier, bringing the oil and water phases together to form a cream.

Character - A description of the aroma of an essential oil.

Chelated/chelation - In the process of chelation, an amino acid is wrapped around the mineral to hide an electrical charge. Minerals carry a negative ion charge, and the body doesn't absorb anything with an electrical charge. When the charge is disguised, the body can absorb and utilize the mineral.

Chemotype – Visually identical plants with significantly different chemical components, resulting in different therapeutic properties.

Citric acid – Citric acid, a naturally occurring plant acid, is found abundantly in lemons (where it was discovered in 1784), and many other fruits including raspberries, black currants, and gooseberries. However, commercial citric acid isn't derived from lemons, or any citrus fruit for that matter because it can't be extracted in a stable form. Instead it's obtained by metabolization of glucose or sucrose by aspergillus niger. In our case, the glucose is derived from certified GMO free corn. It has a sour, acidic taste and is responsible for the tart, sour taste of many unripe fruits. Citric acid is commonly used in the food industry to add tartness to foods and beverages, and in the textile industry to brighten colors.

Cocamidopropyl Betaine – Derived from coconuts. Serves as a gentle surfactant compared to more harsh sulfated surfactants. Cleansing agent.

Cocamidopropylamine Oxide – Derived from coconut oil; produces rich foam. It is a gentle and mild cleansing agent.

Cocos Nucifera (Coconut) Oil - Extracted from the nut meat of ripe coconuts; serves as an excellent moisturizer with high fatty acid content.

Corn syrup solids - Dried corn syrup (derived from corn starch) is referred to as corn syrup solids. It has a relatively low level of sweetness and bland flavor making it useful in blended mixes. Corn syrup solids are added as a flavor enhancer, stabilizer (to reduce product separation during shipping, storage, etc.), and thickener. Corn syrup solids are used in many food applications; baked goods, candy, ice cream, jellies, condiments, powdered sugar, and numerous beverages.

Cryogenic grinding - Cryogenic grinding is a process of mixing nitrogen with an herb or spice to lower the temperature to between 0 and minus 70 degrees F, then grinding the supercooled product. This type of grinding system protects a plant's essential oils and other vital constituents that could be lost during conventional grinding, where temperatures can reach

200 degrees Fahrenheit. Frontier uses cryogenic grinding in order to protect the quality of our herbs and spices.

Cymbopogon Schoenanthus (Lemongrass) Leaf Extract - Derived from the leaves of lemongrass; used as a natural preservative. Lemongrass brightens the complexion.

Dead Sea Salt - Softens the water and provides a gentle, mineral-skin treatment.

Decoction - Decoctions are herbal teas made by boiling herbs in water. Hard or dense plant parts such as roots, barks or seeds with little or no volatile substances are often prepared as decoctions. To make a decoction, add 1 ounce of dried herb to 1 pint of pure water (distilled is best) and place in a glass or other non-reactive container. Cover and place over high heat until water begins to boil. Lower heat and continue to simmer for approximately 15-25 minutes, then cool and strain. Decoctions should be used immediately or refrigerated and used within 2 days.

Decorticated - Decorticating is a term for removing the shell or the pod and the paper thin husk that surrounds cardamom seeds.

Demulcent - A demulcent is a mucilage-rich substance that can be used to coat a mucous membrane with a thin layer that helps to soothe and protect it. When used on the skin, a demulcent is called an emollient. Demulcents are often ingredients in throat products. Plants well known for their demulcent properties include: marshmallow, comfrey, slippery elm, Irish moss, flax seed and licorice.

Dewhiskered - De-Whiskering is the process of removing the small hair-like stem attached to the seed. Whiskers are commonly found in members of the Umbelliferae family such as anise, dill and cumin seeds.

Diffuser - And aromatherapy accessory used to gently disperse essential oils into the air for olfactory benefit.

Diffusion - Diffusion is the spontaneous movement of liquid, gas, or solid particles from an area of high concentration to low concentration. For example, uncapping a bottle of essential oil produces diffusion as the volatile constituents move from the bottle (an area of high concentration) into the environment (an area of low concentration) without being acted upon by heat or pressure. This could also be referred as spontaneous evaporation. Technically, all of the apparatuses used in aromatherapy vaporize or volatilize essential oils because they are acted upon by heat, and/or pressure, to produce fine separated particles or vapor.

Dimethicone - Sand derived raw material; improves lubricity in dry down

Disodium Edta - Derived from sodium chloride; serves as chelating agent.

Distillate - A product of distillation. For example, lavender oil is the distillate of the fresh, blooming lavender plant.

Distillation - The primary method of producing essential oils is through steam distillation. Distillation is an age-old process. While the crude still of the past (almost identical to the simple country "moonshine" still) is now often replaced with modern, stainless steel versions, the process is still basically unchanged. Water is heated to boiling and steam passes through fresh plant material stacked on a rack above the boiling water, causing the cell walls of the plant to break down and release the essential oil. The water and essential oil vapor then pass through a cooler that condenses the steam and the oil into a liquid. The liquid is collected and the oil separates from the water. Most oils are lighter than water and thus collect on the surface of the water where they are siphoned off. Oils heavier than water sink to the bottom of the collector where they are removed. Some stills use "direct," or "water" distillation where the plant material is mixed with boiling water with the same effect.

Eclectic Medicine - Eclectic medicine was a branch of medicine developed in the United States for about a century from the mid-1800s to 1939, when the last Eclectic school of medicine closed. It incorporated the use of herbs and other remedies in alignment with nature and opposed the use of bloodletting, mercury and strong chemicals, which were prevalent at the time. The demise of this branch of medicine occurred when a reform of medical schools, undertaken in the early 1900's, resulted in uniform standards and a curriculum advocated by the AMA (American Medical Association), a strictly science-based model that supported the use of chemical constituents over whole herbs. The reforms gradually took hold and the AMA obtained control of medical education in each state, thus ensuring their system of medicine would be the only legally practiced system allowed. The center of Eclectic education was in Cincinnati, Ohio and the school there was the last to close. Today, the Lloyd Library and Museum in Cincinnati houses many of the papers and books of the Eclectics including the libraries from many of the Eclectic schools.

Emollient - An emollient is a mucilage-rich substance that helps to soothe, soften, smooth and protect the skin. Oils like jojoba are considered emollient to the skin, as are glycerin, lanolin and aloe vera juice. Herbs that have an emollient effect on the skin include: marshmallow, comfrey, slippery elm, flax seed, oats, and chickweed.

Enfleurage - Ancient method for extracting essential oils, commonly used before steam distillation was created. It involves using odorless fats and oils to absorb the oil from the plant material.

Essential Oil - The highly concentrated, volatile, aromatic essences of plants.

Ethical wildcrafting - Ethical wildcrafting is the practice of harvesting plants from the wild in a sustainable manner. Many wild medicinal herb populations are declining due to overharvesting and loss of habitat. Other than ginseng where harvesting of wild plants is regulated by each state, there are no universally accepted regulations for ethically wildcrafted herbs. A number of companies and organizations have developed their own standards for ethical wild harvesting of medicinal herbs. These include criteria such as the percentage of plants that can be harvested in a given population and where and when wild herbs can be harvested.

Ethyl Alcohol - Ethyl alcohol is a plant derived alcohol. It is produced from the fermentation of sugars from plants such as sugarcane, sugar beets or grapes.

Expression - Method of obtaining essential oil from plant material, such as citrus fruit peel. The complete oil is physically forced from the plant material. Also known as cold press extraction.

Extra - The highest, most expensive grade of ylang ylang which is also distilled the shortest length of time. The result is a stronger aroma.

Extraction Method - The method by which essential oils are separated from the plant. Common extraction methods include distillation, expression and solvent extraction.

FDA - Food and Drug Administration. The FDA is a federal agency responsible for protecting public health by guaranteeing the safety, efficacy and security of human and veterinary drugs, foods and cosmetics.

Fannings - Tea is graded by leaf size. Fannings are the very small broken leaves, and are often used for tea bags.

Fixative - A fixative is a substance, often an essential oil, but possibly an herb or animal product, of low volatility that serves to draw together and hold the aromatherapy formula together. Most blends include fixatives, as they will slow the evaporation process and preserve the aromatic qualities. Common essential oil fixatives include vetiver, patchouli, sandalwood, amyris, myrrh and others.

Flower Essences - Flower essences are dilute liquid extracts of various flowers and plants used to treat animals and people, similar to the principles of homeopathy. Flower essence therapy was developed in the 1930's by Dr. Edward Bach, an English physician. Dr. Bach believed that disease was the result of imbalance or negativity at the level of the soul and that flower remedies act to balance these in-harmonies on an emotional and spiritual level. Flower essences are prepared in an exacting way that preserves the essence or energy of the flower. Flower essences are generally used as part of an overall program of health enhancement.

Flush - A flush is the sprouting of new leaves and buds on a tea bush. The number of times a tea plant may flush depends on where it is grown-- with higher, colder regions having only one flush a year; to Sumatra, where the tea plants put out new leaves all year round. Some teas, such as Darjeeling, are graded and sold by flush.

Fold - A term used to designate the strength of vanilla extract according to the amount of vanilla beans used to make the extract. The FDA sets the standard fold strength. Single fold means the extractive matter from 13.35 ounces of vanilla beans in each gallon of liquid. Double fold vanilla contains 26.7 ounces, triple fold, 40.5 ounces, etc. Most vanilla sold at retail is single fold. The higher folds are usually used in food manufacturing.

Fomentation - A fomentation is an herbal compress that is used for applying herbs, in a liquid form, externally to the body. A clean, white cotton cloth is soaked in a liquid herbal preparation such as an herbal tea (infusion), decoction or tincture and then wrung out to remove excess moisture. The cloth is placed on the desired body part, and covered with another cloth to slow drying. The cloth can be reapplied as needed. A fomentation can be warm, cool or can alternate between warm and cool depending on the purpose.

Food Grade - Considered safe for use in food by the Food and Drug Administration.

Fractional Distillation - A distillation method that is interrupted every few hours; the different grades produced are sold separately. This is most commonly used with ylang ylang.

Fragrance - Aroma. Products labeled as fragrances are not pure essential oils. They are derived by synthetic means.

Fumigation - Fumigation is the process of applying a smoke or vapor to a product to destroy pests. At Frontier we use carbon dioxide as a natural fumigant. Unless a botanical is organic, it may have been subjected to chemical fumigants such as methyl bromide. Fumigation does not kill bacteria, only insects and sometimes insect eggs. See also sterilization.

Gas chromatography (GC) - Gas chromatography (GC) is a method of measuring the volatile chemical constituents of a substance. It is one of four objective tests that Frontier uses to determine the quality, identity and purity of every essential oil. GC analysis produces a "fingerprint" of the oil by showing the quantitative presence of each chemical compound. The results can be compared to established standards and reveal oil purity and other information (even the country of origin) which helps validate the oil quality. GC readings that are inconsistent with established standards can be the result of contamination, adulteration, the use of wrong plant parts or species, "off season" harvesting, improper distillation techniques, or product enhancement practices that Frontier finds unacceptable.

GCMS (Gas chromatography/mass spectrometry) – Gas chromatography/mass spectrometry (GCMS) is a method for identifying and analyzing the volatile chemical constituents of a substance. GCMS is a useful tool for analyzing essential oil. GC produces a "fingerprint" of the oil by showing the quantitative presence of each chemical compound. Mass spectrometry identifies each one of those compounds. In order to set our specifications at Frontier, we ran GCMS on each of our oils to identify the chemical components. Then we conducted extensive testing of a variety of oil samples and combined that with extensive review of the scientific literature to develop GC specifications that help us assure that all of our essential oils are authentic, pure, unadulterated and of the highest quality.

GMP (Good Manufacturing Practice) - Good Manufacturing Practices, or GMPs, as they are usually referred to, are a system of standards and processes relating to how a product is made or manufactured. The FDA (Food and Drug Association) publishes, in the <u>Code of Federal Regulations</u>, the GMPs for food and dietary supplements.

GRAS - Generally Recognized as Safe (for human consumption). Foods for which there is a long history of safe use or a general recognition of safety through scientific procedures are considered GRAS by the FDA and not subject to food additive status.

Ginsenosides - Ginseng, known as Ren-sen or "man root" to the Chinese, has been labeled by researchers as an "adaptogen" because it has the intrinsic ability to normalize body functions. The "adaptogenic" effects are thought to be caused by the presence of ginsenosides or tetracyclic terpenoids, the major constituents of ginseng. Researchers have identified 28 different ginsenosides, in varying percentages among the panax species, although 6 (Rb1, Rb2, Rc, Rd, Re, Rg1) are the most significant. The levels vary due to the age of the plant, soil quality, time of harvest, plan part and other environmental factors inherent to the growing region. The precise type and ratio of ginsenosides present can only be determined through HPLC (High Pressure Liquid Chromatography) testing. All parts of the plant may contain ginsenosides; the roots may contain up to 5% but levels are more commonly in the 2-3% range.

Glucose - Plant starch. Humectant. Binding agent.

Glycerin - Glycerin (or glycerine) is a colorless, odorless, viscous, water-soluble liquid with a slightly sweet taste. To avoid it, look for vegetable glycerin on the label. Glycerin is used as a carrier for flavors, a humectant (a substance that promotes retention of moisture) and as an ingredient in baked goods to preserve moisture and prevent staleness. Frontier carries USP-grade Glycerin made from plant sources.

Glycerine (in body care) - A vegetable derived ingredient that serves as a humectant in skin care products by drawing moisture from the environment. It is also used in cosmetic formulations for its smoothing and softening properties.

Glycerol Stearate - A vegetable oil, usually coconut oil derived; serves as a co-emulsifier and helps create a creamy appearance. Also helps to build rich viscosity. Glycerol stearate is lubricious and acts as a humectant by attracting moisture to the skin.

Green tea - Green teas have a grassy, brothy, astringent flavor. Green teas are more widely consumed in Asia. However, with the release of a number of studies on the health benefits of drinking green tea, sales of green tea are growing in the U.S. at over 30%. Green tea is made by first steaming or pan-frying the fresh leaves to prevent the oxidation process that produces black tea. Next the leaves are rolled and then the tea is fired to dry the leaves.

Hydroxypropyltrimonium Chloride - Derived from rubber tree; serves as a natural thickening agent.

Guided minerals - A guided substance is created when transporters such as oxide, gluconate, aspartate, or citrate are added to a chelated substance, further suppressing the electrical charges of the substance. This process, commonly used on minerals, is believed to allow even greater absorption and utilization by the body.

HACCP (Hazard Analysis Critical Control Points) – HACCP is commonly used acronym for the program that defines Hazard Analysis Critical Control Point and is used to describe a program designed to ensure food safety. It is based on identifying the places (Critical Control Points) in a system, starting from receipt of the raw material to the complete assembly of the final product, where chemical, physical or microbiological hazards can enter the process. At each of these points, a plan is put in place to monitor that the defined hazard does not enter the system. Documentation of the program, critical control points and monitoring and corrective actions are all-important parts of a HACCP plan.

HPLC (High Performance Liquid Chromatography) – HPLC (high performance liquid chromatography) is an analytical method used for the separation, identification and quantification of chemical components of various substances. Frontier used HPLC to test various botanicals for adulterants, active or key constituents and to verify identity and quality.

Hahnemann, Dr. Samuel - Dr. Samuel Hahnemann was the founder of homeopathy. While researching the toxicological effects of medicinals in the 1800s, Hahnemann, a German physician and chemist, discovered the concept of "like cures like" also referred to as the "law of similars" or homeopathy. He was considered eccentric for his belief that symptoms were an outward reflection of the body's inner fight to overcome illness; not a manifestation of the illness itself. He also believed in the concept of do no harm and that common practices of the day often caused more harm than good. His concepts included using different potencies during the healing process to allow the body to heal more completely, basing the remedies in liquids (alcohol and water) that are absorbed into the system more readily than tablets and offering only hand-succussed remedies (the remedy is shaken or succussed after each dilution). The results of Hahnemann's studies are published in The Organon of Medicine.

Heat unit (HU) - A heat unit is a measure of the pungency (heat) of a chili pepper. A scale using heat units to measure pungency was developed in the early 1900s by Wilbur Scoville. Scoville also developed a taste test method for rating heat intensity of chilies. Advances in technology have replaced Scoville testing at most companies with <u>HPLC (High Pressure Liquid Chromatography)</u> testing, which separates and measures the level of capsaicin (the chemical responsible for pungency). With HPLC testing, heat intensity is expressed in ASTA units. However, because people are more familiar with the Scoville system, a conversion system has been developed to convert ASTA units to Scoville. (See also <u>Scoville</u>.)

Herbal, Herbalism - Pertaining to natural botanicals and living plants.

Herbal tea - Herbal teas are not really teas in the true sense; they are herbal "infusions" or "tisanes". "True tea" comes from the botanical Camellia sinensis (formerly known as Thea sinensis.) Herbal teas are made by pouring one cup of boiling water over two to three teaspoons of chopped herbs, and steeping for 3 to 5 minutes. They can be made from a variety of botanicals, including spices, roots, leaves, seeds and flowers.

Homeopathy - Homeopathy is a system of healing that aims to stimulate the body's innate healing processes through the administration of minute homeopathic dilutions of specific remedies. Homeopathy uses natural substances from all three realms of nature: plant, mineral and animal. In homeopathy, symptoms are believed to be our bodies attempt to heal itself. Remedies are prescribed in very diluted doses. The same remedies, in higher doses, would produce the symptoms in a healthy person.

Hybrid - Natural or artificially produced plant resulting from the fertilization of one species by another; indicated by 'X' as in lavandula x intermedia or citrus x paradisi.

Hydrosol - Hydrosol, also called hydrolat or floral water, is the name for the water remaining after the steam distillation of an essential oil. A hydrosol is composed mostly of water, with small amounts of the water-soluble parts of the plants being distilled. Because hydrosols contain components that differ from their corresponding essential oils, their uses are not the same. Hydrosols are often used in skin care products and body sprays for their skin-soothing or purifying effects. Because of the very low levels (or even absence) of the more potent and sometimes skin-irritating constituents of the essential oils, hydrosols are very gentle and safe to use on all skin types. Although hydrosols can exist for any distilled essential oil, many are not widely used or available. Some of the more popular hydrosols include rose, lavender, orange blossom, chamomile, neroli, melissa and elderflower waters. One of the problems with true hydrosols is creating a shelf-stable product. Because they are primarily water and do not have naturally occurring preservatives as a component, they do not store for very long. Hydrosols without any preservative listed on the label may be suspect. Products that are not true hydrosols, but rather essential oil mixed with water, with or without the addition of stabilizers and surfactants, are sometimes sold as hydrosols.

Hygroscopic - Hygroscopic refers to a substance that takes up moisture and holds it. Hygroscopic botanicals and minerals such as garlic powder and salt need to be stored in a manner that protects them from humidity or they will clump up and eventually become solid. Anti-caking agents, such as silicon dioxide and calcium stearate and tricalcium phosphate, are added as free-flowing agents to some food products to prevent caking. The only free-flowing agent Frontier uses is silicon dioxide, a natural product that is approved for use by the USDA for use in organic products.

I.U./International Unit - The Dictionary of Scientific Terms defines an I.U. or International Unit as: "A quantity of vitamins, hormones, antibiotics, or other biological that produces a specific internationally accepted biological effect." I.U. is most often seen as a measure of potency of vitamin E.

Infusion - Infusions are liquid preparations made by extracting herbs with either hot or cold water. Infusions are usually used for the more delicate plant parts such as the leaves and flowers. Cold-water infusions are sometimes used for herbs with high volatile oil content. To prepare a cold-water infusion, add the herbs directly to the cool water and let steep in the refrigerator for 6-12 hours, strain. To make a hot-water infusion, place 2-3 t. of dried herbs in a glass or ceramic container. Pour 1 cup of boiling water over the herbs, cover tightly, and let steep for 5 to 10 minutes, then strain To make a stronger infusion, let the mixture steep until cool before straining.

Insoluble - Unable to be dissolved in a liquid such as water.

Irradiation - Frontier does not use irradiation to sterilize products due to our concerns for quality and safety. Irradiation is a food sanitizing and preservation method that uses high-energy ionizing radiation from gamma rays (cobalt 60) or high-energy electrons commonly know as x-rays to reduce the number of microorganisms present in food. This process does not completely eliminate microorganisms or protect treated food from future contamination (due to poor handling practices), but it kills the majority of offensive bacteria in foods. It cannot rejuvenate food that has "passed its prime," by altering signals that indicate spoilage, but it can extend the shelf life of many foods if it is done when food is in prime condition. Irradiation is used routinely in approximately 40 countries. The FDA, Food and Agriculture Organization, and World Health organization oversee all aspects of domestic and international food irradiation including decisions on what foods can be irradiated, the radiation dose that can be used, and the labeling of treated products. In the early 1980s, the FDA approved the use of irradiation on spices and dried vegetable seasonings in the U.S. Foods that have been irradiated must be labeled as being treated with radiation or have the radura (the international symbol for irradiated food) on the label. However, foods that use an irradiated ingredient do not have to note this on the label. Spices on your grocery store shelf are probably not irradiated, but you may ingest irradiated spices as part of your salad dressing, frozen dinner or other prepared food.

Jasminum Officinale Absolute - An absolute derived from freshly picked jasmine flowers. Rich, exotic-floral aroma. Sensuous and calming.

Kosher certified - To be Kosher-certified, a Kosher certification company must inspect the production process from start to finish, checking every conveyor belt, container and piece of processing and packaging machinery to ensure that nothing non-kosher gets into the food. Most Frontier spices and seasonings are kosher. This is noted in the information for individual items.

Lauramidoyl Insulin - Derived from an inulin moiety (chicory) and a lauryl moiety (from coconut oil or palm kernel oil); functions as a straight chain polysaccharide natural emulsifier.

Limbic System - A part of the brain that regulates emotion, appetite, and survival responses.

Lipid - A fat or fat-like substance insoluble in water and soluble in organic solvents.

Lung Ching - Another name for Dragonwell tea.

Maceration - The extraction of substances from a plant by steeping in a fixed oil.

Magnesium - Magnesium is a mineral essential to human health. It is second to calcium in concentration present in the body with 60% of that in the bones, 26% in the muscle and rest in soft tissues such as the brain, heart, liver and kidneys. Foods rich in magnesium are legumes, seeds, nuts, whole grains, tofu and leafy green vegetables. Food processing removes much of the magnesium from foods and thus many Americans who eat a diet high in refined foods are deficient in magnesium.

Magnesium is critical to many cellular functions such as energy production, reproduction of cells and protein formation.

Magnesium Stearate – Stearic acid. Bulking agent.

Maltodextrin – Maltodextrin is a carbohydrate classified GRAS (Generally Recognized As Safe) by the FDA. It has a bland flavor with little or no sweetness and dissolves in hot or cold water. The organic maltodextrin Frontier uses is made from organic tapioca starch and water. There is no corn involved in its manufacture. We typically use maltodextrin to help evenly distribute the flavors of blends.

Mass Spectroscopy (MS) – A lab technique used to identify components in a substance by determining their atomic or molecular masses.

Melissa Officinalis (Balm Mint) Leaf Extract – Derived from lemon balm leaves; used as a natural preservative. Lemon balm brightens the complexion.

Menstruum - Menstruum is the solvent used to extract a plant's constituents. Water and alcohol, alone or in combination, are the most often used solvents, depending on the solubility of the herb's constituents. Glycerin is sometimes used as a solvent instead of alcohol to make a glycerite, or alcohol-free extract. Other solvents or menstruum include vinegar or acetic acid (used to make herb vinegars) and vegetable oil.

Microcrystalline cellulose - Microcrystalline cellulose is naturally occurring cellulose that has been purified. It is found in fruits and vegetables. Commercially produced MCC is isolated from wood pulp, since this is the most economical source. The cellulose is washed, filtered, re-slurried and then spray-dried into its final form. It is considered a safe, stable ingredient and is used extensively in the pharmaceuticals and in foods. At Frontier, we use it in some products such as chili powder, salt and seasoning mixes as an anti-caking agent.

Milk Powder - From whole dried organic milk. Contains potent skin-nourishing proteins, acids, and vitamins.

Modified food starch - Modified food starch is manufactured by treating starch (usually corn based) with chemicals to breakdown the starch into specific length chains of molecules. This process produces more desirable and useful characteristics such as improved solubility, acid stability and texture. Modified food starch is used in foods as a thickener, binder and stabilizer. It also gives food a desirable mouthfeel.

Monosodium glutamate (MSG) - No Frontier products have MSG added to them. MSG is the sodium salt of glutamic acid. When MSG is ingested, the body converts it almost immediately to glutamate. Glutamate is an amino acid (the building blocks of proteins) and is found in almost all plant and animal tissue. Glutamic acid is present in significant amounts in high protein foods. The human body also produces glutamic acid and stores up to four pounds (in a 150-pound adult) for use in making human protein. There are two forms of glutamate: "bound" and "free". Bound glutamate is linked to other amino acids to form protein molecules. Free glutamate is the single amino acid, glutamate. Both forms occur naturally in our food supply. Unfortunately, some people have allergic reactions to free glutamate.

Mucilage – Mucilage – Mucilage is composed of complex polysaccharides. It is present in a variety of plants. Some of those with large amounts of mucilage include: marshmallow, flax seeds, purslane, chia seeds, and oats (as in oatmeal). It's generally pretty tasteless but has a slimy feel when it comes into contact with water. Mucilage has demulcent properties, and mucilage-rich herbs are used throughout the body for their soothing benefits. (See also demulcent.)

NOP (National Organic Program) – The National Organic Program is responsible for developing, implementing, and administering an organic system of agriculture and the handling and labeling of organic products in accordance with the organic regulations in Title 7, Part 205 of the Code of Federal Regulations. The regulations contained in the code are based on the Organic Foods Production Act of 1990, passed by Congress. A National Organic Standards Board (NOSB) was established by the Act to "assist in the development of standards for substances to be used in organic production" and to "provide recommendations to the Secretary regarding implementation" of the act'. The NOSB is comprised of 15 members, serving five-year terms and representing difference interested sectors including consumer, farmer, process, certifiers, retailers, environmentalists and scientists. The Board solicits input from the public, holds hearings and makes recommendations to the USDA on the organic rules. If approved by the USDA, these rules are subject to the usual review and approval process before becoming official.

Natural - There is no legal U.S. definition for "natural," and neither the FDA nor the USDA has rules regarding the term. Unlike the USDA-regulated term "organic," the designation "natural" can be applied to products at the unregulated discretion of manufacturers.

Natural flavor - The United States Code of Federal Regulations (21 CFR 101.22, and 21 CFR 182.10) gives the following definition: "The term 'natural flavor or natural flavoring means the essential oil, oleoresin, essence or extractive, protein hydrolysate, distillate, or any product of roasting, heating or enzymolysis, which contains the flavoring constituents derived from a spice, fruit or fruit juice, vegetable or vegetable juice, edible yeast, herbs, bark, bud, root, leaf or similar plant material, meat, seafood, poultry, eggs, dairy products or fermentation products thereof, whose significant function in food is flavoring rather than nutritional. Natural flavors include the natural essence or extractives obtained from plants listed in sections 182.10, 182.20, 182.40, and 182.50 and part 184 of this chapter, and the substances listed in section 172.510 of this chapter." Frontier follows the CFR definition.

Neat - A "neat" drop refers to a drop of liquid that is unmixed, or undiluted. Generally applies to the act of applying an essential oil to the body undiluted. Since dilution is nearly always recommended, using oils neat is very uncommon.

Olfactory - Of, relating to or connected with the sense of smell.

Oolong tea - Oolong (English) or Wu Long (Chinese pinyin translation) tea is a partially oxidized tea, and has flavor characteristics of both green and black teas. The fresh leaves are withered for one to two days, then rolled to release enzymes (needed for the next step). Then the tea leaves are allowed to oxidize, although for a shorter period than for black tea, and the process is stopped before it is completed. The tea is fired (heated) to prevent further oxidation and to dry the tea. Oolong teas can vary significantly in flavor depending on when the oxidation process is interrupted, having more of a green tea character if interrupted early in the process, and more black tea character the longer oxidation continues.

Optical rotation – Optical rotation is one of the objective tests performed by Frontier to determine the purity of every essential oil. A sensitive scientific instrument (polarimeter) measures the degree a light ray bends when it is passed through a column of oil. The reading is compared to established standards; significant deviation from the standard may indicate impurities and give cause for further investigation.

Orange Pekoe (OP) – Tea is graded by leaf size. Orange Pekoe is a full leaf tea with no buds.

Organic – Organic is a growing and processing method that helps protect the health of people, plants, animals, and the environment. Organic food is produced by farmers who use renewable resources and conserve soil and water to enhance environmental quality for future generations.

Organic foods are produced without most conventional pesticides, fertilizers made with synthetic ingredients, bioengineering or ionizing irradiation. Before a product can be labeled as organic, a USDA approved certifier must approve the growing, handling and labeling of the product to insure that it complies with all organic regulations.

Organic Foods Production Act of 1990 - The Organic Foods Production Act of 1990 was a landmark bill for organic agriculture. Many groups petitioned Congress to establish a national law to insure uniformity of regulations, inspire consumer confidence in a single organic label, make it easier to market certified organic products overseas and to obtain ingredients certified organic overseas. At the time of the law's passing, there were local, regional, state and national organizations certifying farmers and processors to their own standards. Internationally, each certification group had to establish reciprocity in order to accept the other's certification. Farmers often were forced to obtain certification from multiple agencies – an expensive and time-consuming process. The Act provided for the basis for the organic regulations listed in the Code of Federal Regulations.

Organic certification - The USDA has established rules under the National Organic Program that regulate the growing, handling, labeling and certification of organic food sold in the U.S.

Organoleptic - Organoleptic refers to the sensory properties of a substance, such as taste, color, odor and feel. Organoleptic testing involves inspection through tasting, feeling, smelling and visual examination of a substance.

Oxidize - To react with oxygen, usually causing rapid degradation or deterioration.

Paraffin - Paraffin is a synthetic wax like substance made of solid hydrocarbons distilled from petroleum or from the oil of distilled shale. It is a translucent, virtually odorless material ranging from colorless to white in appearance, and having a slightly greasy texture. Paraffin is graded and sold according to its melting point which ranges between 120 and 200 degrees Fahrenheit, and its color. It is commonly used in candle making, paper coating, lipstick, and for sealing jars of food and is virtually insoluble in water, and alcohol.

Potassium Sorbate - Plant derived ingredient; functions as a toxic free preservative.

Potherb - This is an antiquated English term for any plant that is cooked and eaten as a green. Plants such as spinach or kale would qualify as potherbs. Oftentimes, medicinal herbs were also potherbs, with the stems and leaves picked when the plants are young, then boiled and eaten as a green vegetable or used to flavor soups or grains. The first potherbs to be available in the spring where the wild herbs, which start to grow before garden greens could even be planted. So these wild potherbs were prized, especially after a long winter, because they provided nutrients and fresh flavor to the remnants of winter fare. Many of the herbs were also considered spring tonics, helping to fortify a winter-drained body, cleanse the blood and invigorate. Europeans who emigrated carried their wild potherbs with them for planting in their new gardens. These hardy herbs often became weeds in their new locations when they escaped cultivation.

Some examples of wild potherbs are nettles, dandelion, cleavers, sorrel, chickweed and lamb's quarters.

Propylene glycol – A carrier used in flavors. Some suppliers use this carrier, we request that ours do not.

Prunus Amygdalus Dulcis (Sweet Almond) Oil – High in oleic and linoleic acids. Similar to apricot kernel but slightly more lubricity and glide. Probably the best choice for most massage applications. Appropriate for dry skin, massage and bath.

Prunus Armeniaca (Apricot) Kernel Oil – Provides a medium thickness, glide and lubricity. Use in higher amounts for standard massage, less amounts for friction and heat building massage. Appropriate for combination skin, massage, moisturizing bath oil, after shower nourishing skin care oil.

Prussic acid – Many fruits, nuts, seeds, legumes and pasture type grasses that are a daily part of human and animal diets contain naturally occurring cyanogenic glycosides such as amygdalin, which when ingested, break down into three substances; sugar, cyanide (prussic acid), and benzaldehyde. Benzaldehyde is the substance used as a flavoring and fragrance material. It has an almond or cherry taste, and an almond-like aroma. The kernel of almonds, apricots, plums, peaches, contains prussic acid, although the fruit is entirely unaffected. The kernels of these fruits are used to make almond essential oil. The oil produced from these pits intended for food use is treated to remove prussic acid, and is designated as FFPA (free from prussic acid). The Code of Federal Regulations (21 CFR 582.20) states that prussic acid-free bitter almond oil is considered GRAS (generally recognized as safe) as a food flavoring.

Pu-erh Tea - Pu-erh is a "composted" tea produced in Yunnan province of China. The freshly picked tea is fired then placed in piles and monitored to maintain proper temperature and moisture during the aging process. Pu-erh is a speciality tea with a strong, earthy flavor.

Pycnogenol - Pycnogenol is a registered trademark of Horphag Research, LTD. It is a natural plant extract obtained from the bark of European grown *Pinus maritima* (pine trees), Pycnogenol contains proanthocyanidins, the compounds responsible for the antioxidant properties of the extract. Proanthocyanidins or flavonoids are the plant pigments responsible for the deep blue-red color of many berries including grapes and hawthorn berries. They are also present in cypress bark, Ceylon and cassia cinnamon bark, and many other trees of the Coniferae family.

QAI - Quality Assurance International is a USDA-approved organic certification agency. They have been Frontier's organic certifier for many years. QAI is responsible for inspecting and reviewing our procedures, products, labeling and practices to insure that we are in compliance with all organic regulations.

Qi - Qi or Ch'i (pronounced chee), is a Traditional Chinese Medicine (TCM) term that refers to the vital energy in the body. Qi is at the very heart of the TCM system, it is the invisible force that animates life energy taking shape as matter. Qi comes into the body from the air taken in through the lungs and from the foods we eat. When Qi is depleted, a person will feel tired, weak, clammy, apathetic and unable to fight off invasions of disease. When Qi is strong, a person will feel energetic, strong and vigorous with a high resistance level. Qi should move freely in the body and should be balanced in order to maintain health and well-being.

Radura - The radura is the internationally recognized symbol for irradiated food. All foods that have been irradiated that are sold in the U.S. must either bear this symbol or include wording on the label stating that they have been irradiated.

Raw Food - Though there isn't an official definition for this term, it is generally accepted that a food can be considered raw if it has not been heated above 115 degrees Fahrenheit and has not been frozen.

Refractive index - Refractive index testing is one of four objective testing procedures Frontier uses to determine the quality of every essential oil. A refractometer is used to measure the velocity of a light ray passing through an essential oil. (Light behaves differently depending upon the density of the material it is passing through.) The reading is compared to established literature; deviations are indicative of adulteration.

Retinyl Palmitate (Vitamin A) - Derived from palm kernel oil. Adds skin-nourishing properties to the product, aids in dry skin treatment, essential for growth and maintenance of bones, glands, teeth, nails and hair.

Rosmarinus Officinalis (Rosemary) Leaf Extract - Derived from the leaves of rosemary; used as a natural preservative.

Rubbed - This term, as used in "rubbed sage," refers to a process by which leaves are literally rubbed — by hand or by machine — through a screen until broken into small pieces. This releases the herb's essential oils and heightens its flavor and aroma qualities when used in cooking. The term originates from cooks rubbing leaves of herbs between their fingers as they add them during cooking.

Rubefacient - substances for external application that cause redness of the skin through dilation of the capillaries, which allows for increased blood circulation, resulting in a warming sensation.

Sachet - Sachets are powdered or very small fragrant materials (such as lavender, peppermint, and roses) enclosed in scraps of cloth, cotton drawstring tea bags, or even greeting cards, and heat sealable tea bags. The material is stitched or glued along the outer edges to contain the blend. A fixative helps the sachet retain its scent. Sachets can be used to scent linens and clothes as favors at weddings or parties, or if made with decorative materials, adorning on your desk.

Scoville heat unit - In the early 1900s pharmacist Wilbur Scoville developed a methodology and scale to measure the pungency (heat level) of chili peppers. The system involves a taste test of pepper extract, and a comparison of the results against a standardized scale. To create the extract, peppers are soaked in alcohol for approximately 24 hours to draw out the capsaicin. A specified amount of the pepper extract is then added to sweetened water. The solution is diluted repeatedly until the hotness of the pepper extract is barely detectable. A heat unit rating is then assigned based upon the dilution ratio. For example, a Scoville rating of 20,000 hu for a chili pepper would indicate that it took 20,000 times the volume of sweetened water before the pepper extract was barely detectable. With advances in technology, the Scoville organoleptic testing procedure has been replaced at most companies with HPLC (High Pressure Liquid Chromatography). The American Trade Association (ASTA) supports the use of HPLC testing. With the use of this testing method, heat level is expressed in ASTA units. However, because people are more familiar with the Scoville system, a conversion system has been developed to convert ASTA units to Scoville units.

Sea Salt - Purified, simple sodium chloride isolated from seawater. Creates a buoyant, skin-softening bath water.

Sebaceous Glands - Present in the dermis. Open to the surface at pores located in the epidermis. Produces sebum (oil).

Sebum - The oily substance produced by the sebaceous glands which function to lubricate the skin and seal moisture into the cells. The level of sebum production determines whether your skin is normal, dry or oily.

Shelf life - Shelf life of botanicals can vary significantly with each product depending on plant part and size. Storage conditions also impact shelf life with heat, light, moisture and air all affecting the quality of the botanical. Botanicals and essential oils do not have a date when they go bad, rather the quality gradually declines over time. Some general guidelines on when to replace well stored botanicals and essential oils are:

- *Whole spices and herbs*
  - Leaves and flowers: 1 to 2 years
  - Seeds and barks: 2 to 3 years
  - Roots: 3 years
- *Ground spices and herbs*
  - Leaves and flowers: 1 year
  - Seeds and barks: 1 year
  - Roots: 2 years

- *Teas*
  - Black, green, white and oolong: 1 year
  - *Essential Oils*
  - Citrus and pine oils: 1 year
  - Other essential oils: 3 to 5 years

Silicon Dioxide (SiO2) - Silicon dioxide is an oxide of silica, the most abundant mineral in the earth's crust and found in as sand or quartz. Silicon dioxide is found naturally in some plant-based foods. As an additive to foods, it is used as a free-flowing agents in powders and hygroscopic (water attracting) substances.

Simmondsia Chinensis (Jojoba) Oil - Light-textured, pH balanced liquid wax pressed from the jojoba nut. Mimics natural pH and function of the skin's own sebum.

Smudging - Smudging is a traditional method of burning herbs or wands of herbs called smudge sticks and bathing oneself or an object in the smoke to clear away negative influences and restore balance. Many people like to smudge their home, office or space to change the energy of that area.

Sodium Bicarbonate - Naturally derived from minerals. Cleansing agent.

Sodium Borate - A naturally occurring mined desert mineral, sodium borate has a mild, soap-like cleansing action.

Sodium Carbonate - Sodium carbonate, water, and carbon dioxide.

Sodium Carboxymethyl Betaglucan - Derived from yeast cell wall; protects against UV-A induced oxidative stress, restores skin function, promotes cell renewal and enhances skin's self-protection mechanism.

Sodium Chloride - Derived from nature. Helps lift away old, dead cells while soothing and softening the skin.

Sodium Cocoyl Isethionate - Coconut-derived. Cleansing agent.

Sodium Hydroxymethylglycinate - Produced from sodium chloride; serves as a safe, broad spectrum, paraben-free preservative system.

Sodium Myreth Sulfate - Derived from coconut oil; produces rich foam and builds viscosity. Excellent cleanser that is compatible with all skin types.

Soluble - Able to be dissolved in a liquid such as water.

Steam Distillation - A method of essential oil extraction using steam.

Sterilization - Sterilization is the process of killing microbes on a product. Sterilizing a product also kills insects and insects eggs (fumigation). Herbs and spices are sterilized by one of three methods - heat, chemical or irradiation. Heat sterilization is used on some hard spices such as peppercorns. Chemical sterilization is done with ethylene oxide. In the U.S.,treatment of spices with ionizing radiation is allowed, however such spices must be so labeled. See also radura and irradiation.

Sun Tea - Sun tea is tea brewed slowly by the sun. To make, put four teaspoons of tea per quart in a glass jar, filled with cool water, stir and place in the sun for six hours. Strain and serve or refrigerate.

Synthetic - An artificially produced substance designed to imitate that which occurs naturally.

TCM (Traditional Chinese Medicine) - TCM is a complete system of natural health care that has been used for several thousand years and is still used today to treat one-quarter of the earth's population. It is very different in theory and practice from Western health care. TCM is based on the concept of balance of the vital energy, Qi (chee) that flows freely through the body of a healthy being. Living in harmony with nature and striving for moderation and balance in all things are core principles. Disease is the result of disruption of this balance. The practitioner's role is patient-based, rather than ailment-based as in Western medicine, so that a remedy is not prescribed based so much on the condition as it is on the patient and their constitution. Components of TCM include diet, exercise, acupuncture, herbs and massage.

Cacao Butter - Cocoa beans.This natural butter melts into skin at body temperature and provides rich emollience and moisture retention.

Tincture - A tincture is a stable liquid preparation that contains an herb's desired constituents. It's made using a solvent or menstruum tailored to dissolve the maximum amount of the chemical components of the whole herb. Once the components are extracted, the herb and solvent mixture is pressed to remove the liquid from the solids (marc). The resulting liquid is filtered and then stored in dark bottles in a cool place. Tinctures are a good way to preserve an herb over several years, and they're convenient to carry and use.

Orange Pekoe - Tea leaves are graded by size. Tippy golden flowery orange pekoe is a full leaf tea with many golden buds.

Tisane - Tisane is another name for herbal tea (as opposed to black or green tea). The term originated in France and is derived from the Latin term "ptisana".

Tocopheryl Acetate (Vitamin E) – Powerful and skin-supporting. Safe and natural preservative.

Vanilla Extract – The FDA has a standard of identity for vanilla extract. To be called an extract, it must contain at least 35% alcohol by volume. If there is less than 35% alcohol, the product must be labeled a flavor.

Viscosity – Pertaining to the thickness or thinness of a liquid, it especially relates to the speed at which an essential oil pours from the bottle. An example would be vetiver, having a high viscosity, pours extremely slowly from the bottle.

Vitamin E – Vitamin E is an essential nutrient, meaning that it must be provided by the diet because the body cannot manufacture it. Vitamin E food sources include some vegetable oils, nuts and whole grains (soy is one of the most common natural sources). Tocopherols are naturally occurring substances, which exhibit vitamin E activity. Alpha tocopherol, thought to be the most active form of vitamin E, is commonly found in supplement form.

WONF - WONF is short for "with other natural flavors." The term is used when an extract or flavoring is made with natural ingredients other than the characterizing flavor ingredient. So for instance if a natural strawberry flavor included other natural fruit flavors, it would be labeled as WONF.

White tea - White teas are a type of green tea made from the unopened leaf buds. It is the least processed of the teas and has a light, grassy, very mild flavor. The fresh picked leaves are immediately steamed to prevent any oxidation and then fired to dry them. The term "white tea" refers to the whitish cast of the tea that comes from the silky white hairs on the tightly closed leaf buds of the tea.

Wild - Growing spontaneously, not cultivated

Wildcrafted - herbs harvested in the wild rather than cultivated.

Xantham Gum - Xantham gum is a natural gum produced by a pure culture fermentation of a starch, typically glucose or sucrose, by Xanthomonas *campestris* bacterium. In the food industry it is used to thicken, suspend, emulsify and stabilize products. It is also used as a substitute for gluten in baked goods. Xantham is a unique gum in respect to its stability under a wide range of temperatures and pH, and is considered GRAS by the USDA.

Yield - The amount of essential oil extracted from a plant.

Ginger Root Extract - Derived from the roots of ginger; used as a natural preservative. Ginger is warming and activating.

References

American Cancer Society

https://www.cancer.org/cancer/esophagus-cancer/about/key-statistics.html

WebMD

https://www.webmd.com/heartburn-gerd/news/20111012/barretts-esophagus-may-be-less-risky-than-thought#1

AARP

https://www.aarp.org/health/conditions-treatments/info-2017/foods-help-acid-reflux-fd.html

American Journal of Forensic Medicine and Pathology

https://journals.lww.com/amjforensicmedicine/Abstract/2007/06000/Barrett_Esophagus_and_Unexpected_Death.13.aspx

NCBI - The National Center for Biotechnology Information

https://www.ncbi.nlm.nih.gov/pmc/articles/PMC4113043/

National Center For Health Statistics

https://www.cdc.gov/nchs/index.htm

Heathline

https://www.healthline.com/health/barretts-esophagus-diet#takeaway

The MAYO Clinic

DrAxe

World Incidence of Esophageal Cancer

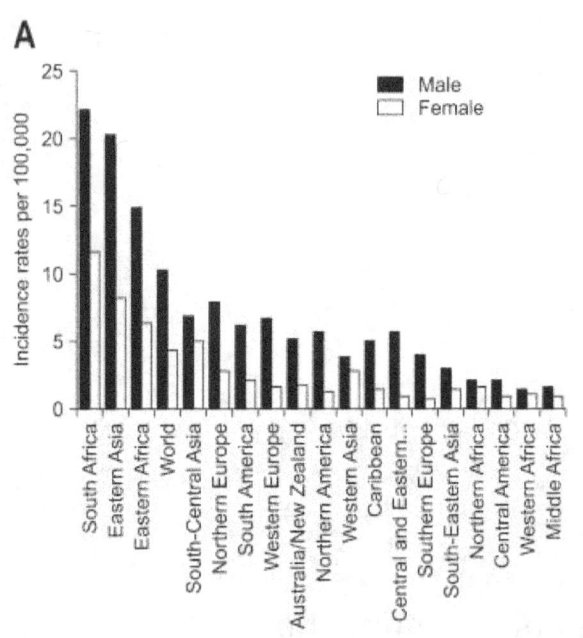
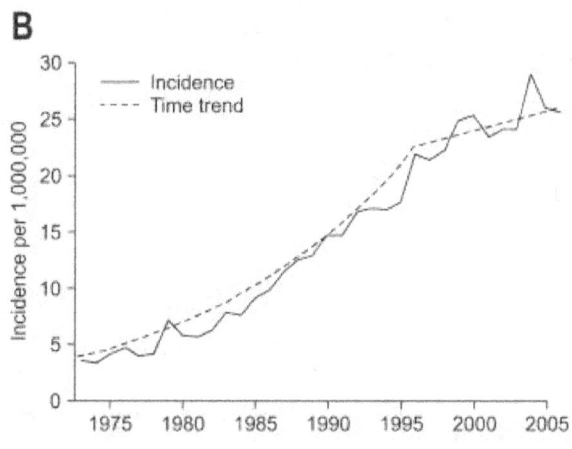

Fig. 1

(A) World age-standardized incidence rates of esophageal cancer per 100,000 population. Estimates derived from Cancer Research UK statistics (Ferlay J, *et al*. GLOBOCAN 2008 v1.2, cancer incidence and mortality worldwide).[14] (B) Relative change in the incidence of esophageal adenocarcinoma (1973 to 2006). With permission from Pohl H, *et al*. Cancer Epidemiol Biomarkers Prev 2010;19:1468–1470.[15]

www.ingramcontent.com/pod-product-compliance
Lightning Source LLC
Chambersburg PA
CBHW081206280526
45787CB00006B/2342